Virtual Medical Office

for

Young: Kinn's The Medical Assistant,
11th Edition

Virtual Medical Office

for

Young: Kinn's The Medical Assistant, 11th Edition

Study Guide prepared by

Tracie Fuqua, BS, CMA(AAMA)
Program Director
Medical Assistant Program
Wallace State Community College
Hanceville, Alabama

Textbook by

Alexandra Patricia Young-Adams, BBA, RMA, CMA(AAMA)

Adjunct Instructor
Everest College, Arlington Midcities Campus
Arlington, Texas

Professional Writer
Grand Prairie, Texas

Formerly
Director of Admissions
Parker College of Chiropractic
Dallas, Texas

Formerly
Program Director
Medical Assisting/HIM Programs
Ultrasound Diagnostic School
Irving, Texas

Deborah B. Proctor, EdD, RN
Professor and
Medical Assisting Program Director
Butler County Community College
Butler, Pennsylvania

Software developed by

Wolfsong Informatics, LLC
Tucson, Arizona

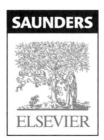

SAUNDERS

ELSEVIER

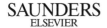

3251 Riverport Lane
Maryland Heights, Missouri 63043

VIRTUAL MEDICAL OFFICE FOR
YOUNG: KINN'S THE MEDICAL ASSISTANT
ELEVENTH EDITION
Copyright © 2011, 2007 by Saunders, an imprint of Elsevier Inc.

ISBN: 978-1-4377-2405-9

Notice

Knowledge and best practice in this field are constantly changing. As new research and experience broaden our knowledge, changes in practice, treatment and drug therapy may become necessary or appropriate. Readers are advised to check the most current information provided (i) on procedures featured or (ii) by the manufacturer of each product to be administered, to verify the recommended dose or formula, the method and duration of administration, and contraindications. It is the responsibility of the practitioner, relying on their own experience and knowledge of the patient, to make diagnoses, to determine dosages and the best treatment for each individual patient, and to take all appropriate safety precautions. To the fullest extent of the law, neither the Publisher nor the Authors assumes any liability for any injury and/or damage to persons or property arising out or related to any use of the material contained in this book.

ISBN: 978-1-4377-2405-9

Acquisitions Editor: Susan Cole
Developmental Editor: Karen Baer
Publishing Services Manager: Gayle May
Project Manager: Stephen Bancroft

Printed in the United States of America

Last digit is the print number: 9 8 7 6 5 4 3 2

Table of Contents

Reviewers

Sandra L. Alexander, BAS, CMA(AAMA)
Medical Assisting Program Director/Coordinator
Health/Legal Studies
El Centro College
Dallas, Texas

Cynthia Y. Hill, MBA, BS, CHI, COLT (AMT), CPT, CEHRS
Professor
Allied Health
Cuyahoga Community College
Highland Heights, Ohio

Deborah S. Ginbey, RN, MSN, MA
Instructor
Nursing
Wayland Baptist University
San Antonio, Texas

Stacey F. Wilson, MT/PBT (ASCP), CMA(AAMA), MHA
Program Chair, Medical Assistant
Medical Assisting
Cabarrus College of Health Sciences
Concord, North Carolina

Getting Started

■ LOGIN AND ENROLLMENT INSTRUCTIONS

Please check with your instructor prior to registering to verify whether you are required to enroll in the instructor's *Virtual Medical Office* course on Evolve. If so, your instructor will provide you with your course ID and you will use the steps under **Instructor-Led Course** on the following page.

SELF-STUDY COURSE

1. To access your Virtual Medical Office, please visit http://evolve.elsevier.com/Kinn/.
2. Select the **Simulations—VMO** tab and click **Register for These Simulations** to begin the one-time-only registration process.
3. Select **I already have an Access code** and enter the code located on the inside front cover of this study guide exactly as it appears.
4. Click **Register**.
5. If you already have an Evolve account or have previously requested products from Evolve, provide your case-sensitive username and password in the Returning User area and click **Login**. If you do not have an Evolve account, provide your desired password for the account in the New User area and click **Continue**. Provide the required profile information and click **Continue**.
6. Read the Registered User Agreement. Check **Yes, I accept this agreement** and then click **Submit**.
7. A screen confirming your enrollment will appear. Click **My Home**.
8. This product will be added to your Evolve account under the My Content area located on the left-hand side of the Evolve homepage. Click to expand the **Simulations—VMO** heading and then click the link titled **Young: Kinn's The Medical Assistant, Eleventh Edition**.
9. Click **Simulations—VMO** to access your activities.
10. Your case-sensitive account information will be emailed to you. Please note your account information. If needed, you can request your account information at any time by clicking on the **I forgot my login information** link on the Evolve homepage.
11. Please bookmark this page (http://evolve.elsevier.com/student) to easily log in and access your *Virtual Medical Office* in the future.

1

INSTRUCTOR-LED COURSE

1. Go to http://evolve.elsevier.com/enroll.
2. Enter the **Course ID** provided to you by your instructor and click the arrow button.
3. Verify that the course information is correct and check **Yes, this is my course**.
4. Select **I already have an Access code** and enter the code located on the inside front cover of this study guide exactly as it appears.
5. Click **Register**.
6. If you already have an Evolve account or have previously requested products from Evolve, provide your case-sensitive username and password in the Returning User area and click **Login**. If you do not have an Evolve account, provide your desired password for the account in the New User area and click **Continue**. Provide the required profile information and click **Continue**.
7. Read the Registered User Agreement. Check **Yes, I accept this agreement** and click **Submit**.
8. A screen confirming your enrollment will appear. Click **Get Started** or **My Home**.
9. This product will be added to your Evolve account under the My Content area located on the left-hand side of the Evolve homepage. Click to expand the **Simulations—VMO** heading and then click **Young: Kinn's The Medical Assistant, Eleventh Edition**.
10. Click **Course Documents** and then click **Simulations—VMO** to access your activities.
11. Your case-sensitive account information will be emailed to you. Please note your account information. If needed, you can request your account information at any time by clicking on **I forgot my login information** on the Evolve homepage.
12. Please bookmark this page (http://evolve.elsevier.com/student) to easily log in and access your *Virtual Medical Office* in the future.

■ SUPPORT INFORMATION

Visit the Evolve Support Portal at http://evolvesupport.elsevier.com to access the Evolve Knowledge Base, Downloads, and Support Ticket System. Live Evolve Support is also available 24/7 by calling 1-800-401-9962.

GETTING SET UP

■ **TECHNICAL REQUIREMENTS**

To use an Evolve Online Product, you will need access to a computer that is connected to the Internet and equipped with web browser software that supports frames. For optimal performance, it is recommended that you have speakers and use a high-speed Internet connection. Dial-up modems are not recommended for *Virtual Medical Office*.

WINDOWS®

Windows PC
Windows XP, Windows Vista™
Pentium® processor (or equivalent) @ 1 GHz (Recommend 2 GHz or better)
800 x 600 screen size
Thousands of colors
Soundblaster 16 soundcard compatibility
Stereo speakers or headphones
Internet Explorer (IE) version 6.0 or higher
Mozilla Firefox version 2.0 or higher

MACINTOSH®

Mozilla Firefox version 2.0 or higher

■ **WEB BROWSERS**

Supported web browsers include Microsoft Internet Explorer (IE) version 6.0 or higher and Mozilla Firefox version 2.0 or higher.

If you use America Online® (AOL) for web access, you will need AOL version 4.0 or higher, and one of the browsers listed above. Earlier versions of AOL and Internet Explorer will not run the course properly and you will have difficulty accessing many features.

For best results with AOL:
- Connect to the Internet using AOL version 4.0 or higher.
- Open a private chat within AOL. (This allows the AOL client to remain open, without asking if you wish to disconnect while minimized.)
- Minimize AOL.
- Launch one of the recommended browsers.

■ SCREEN SETTINGS

For best results, your computer monitor resolution should be set at a minimum of 800 x 600. The number of colors displayed should be set to "thousands or higher" (High Color or 16 bit) or "millions of colors" (True Color or 24 bit).

WINDOWS

1. From the **Start** menu, select **Settings**, then **Control Panel**.
2. Double-click on the **Display** icon.
3. Click on the **Settings** tab.
4. Under **Screen resolution** use the slider bar to select **800 x 600 pixels**.
5. Access the **Colors** drop-down menu by clicking on the down arrow.
6. Select **High Color (16 bit)** or **True Color (24 bit)**.
7. Click on **Apply**, then **OK**.
8. You may be asked to verify the setting changes. Click **Yes**.
9. You may be asked to restart your computer to accept the changes. Click **Yes**.

MACINTOSH

1. Select the **Monitors** control panel.
2. Select **800 x 600** (or greater) from the **Resolution** area.
3. Select **Thousands** or **Millions** from the **Color Depth** area.

■ SUPPORT INFORMATION

Visit the Evolve Support Portal at http://evolvesupport.elsevier.com to access the Evolve Knowledge Base, Downloads, and Support Ticket System. Live Evolve Support is also available 24/7 by calling 1-800-401-9962.

Enable Cookies

Browser	Steps
Internet Explorer (IE) 6.0 or higher	1. Select **Tools → Internet Options**. 2. Select **Privacy** tab. 3. Use the slider (slide down) to **Accept All Cookies**. 4. Click **OK**. -OR- 3. Click the **Advanced** button. 4. Click the check box next to **Override Automatic Cookie Handling**. 5. Click the **Accept** radio buttons under **First-party Cookies** and **Third-party Cookies**. 6. Click **OK**.
Mozilla Firefox 2.0 or higher	1. Select **Tools → Options**. 2. Select the **Privacy** icon. 3. Click to expand Cookies. 4. Select **Allow sites to set cookies**. 5. Click **OK**.

Set Cache to Always Reload a Page

Browser	Steps
Internet Explorer (IE) 6.0 or higher	1. Select **Tools → Internet Options**. 2. Select **General** tab. 3. Go to the **Temporary Internet Files** and click the **Settings** button. 4. Select the radio button for **Every visit to the page** and click **OK** when complete.
Mozilla Firefox 2.0 or higher	1. Select **Tools → Options**. 2. Select the **Privacy** icon. 3. Click to expand Cache. 4. Set the value to "**0**" in the **Use up to: __ MB of disk space for the cache** field. 5. Click **OK**.

Plug-Ins

 Adobe Acrobat Reader—With the free Acrobat Reader software, you can view and print Adobe PDF files. Many Evolve products offer student and instructor manuals, checklists, and more in this format!

Download at: http://www.adobe.com

 Apple QuickTime—Install this to hear word pronunciations, heart and lung sounds, and many other helpful audio clips within Evolve Online Courses!

Download at: http://www.apple.com

 Adobe Flash Player—This player will enhance your viewing of many Evolve web pages, as well as educational short-form to long-form animation within the Evolve Learning System!

Download at: http://www.adobe.com

 Adobe Shockwave Player—Shockwave is best for viewing the many interactive learning activities within Evolve Online Courses!

Download at: http://www.adobe.com

 Microsoft Word Viewer—With this viewer Microsoft Word users can share documents with those who don't have Word, and users without Word can open and view Word documents. Many Evolve products have testbank, student and instructor manuals, and other documents available for downloading and viewing on your own computer!

Download at: http://www.microsoft.com

Office Tour

Welcome to *Virtual Medical Office*, a virtual office setting in which you can work with multiple patient simulations and also learn to access and evaluate the information resources that are essential for providing high-quality medical assistance.

In the virtual medical office, Mountain View Clinic, you can access the Reception area, Exam Room, Laboratory, Office Manager, and Check Out area, plus a separate room for Billing and Coding.

■ BEFORE YOU START

Make sure you have your textbook nearby when you use *Virtual Medical Office* online. You will want to consult topic areas in your textbook frequently while working online and using this study guide.

■ HOW TO SIGN IN

- After entering the access code included inside this study guide, enter your name on the Medical Assistant identification badge.
- Click on **Start Simulation**.

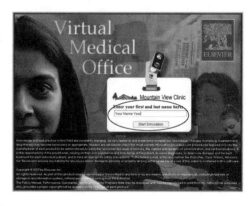

- This takes you to the office map screen. Across the top of this screen is the list of patients available for you to follow throughout their office visit.

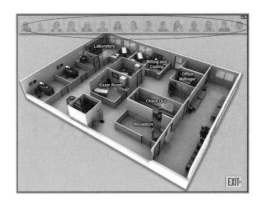

■ PATIENT LIST

1. **Janet Jones (age 50)**—Ms. Jones has sustained an on-the-job injury. She is in pain and impatient. By working with Ms. Jones, students will learn about managing difficult patients, as well as the requirements involved in workers' compensation cases.

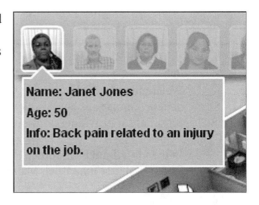

2. **Wilson Metcalf (age 65)**—A Medicare patient, Mr. Metcalf is being seen for multiple symptoms of abdominal pain, nausea, vomiting, and fever. He is seriously ill and might need more specialized care in a hospital setting.

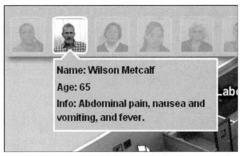

3. **Rhea Davison (age 53)**—An established patient with chronic and multiple symptoms, Ms. Davison does not have medical insurance.

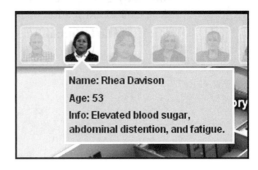

4. **Shaunti Begay (age 15)**—A new patient, Shaunti Begay is a minor who has an appointment for a sports physical. Upon arrival, Shaunti and her family learn that Mountain View Clinic does not participate in their health insurance.

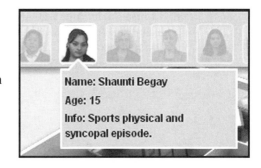

Name: Shaunti Begay
Age: 15
Info: Sports physical and syncopal episode.

5. **Jean Deere (age 83)**—Accompanied by her son, Ms. Deere is an established Medicare patient being evaluated for memory loss and hearing loss.

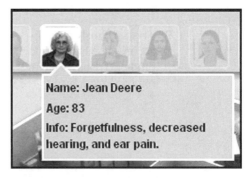

Name: Jean Deere
Age: 83
Info: Forgetfulness, decreased hearing, and ear pain.

6. **Renee Anderson (age 43)**—Ms. Anderson scheduled her appointment for a routine gynecological examination but exhibits symptoms that suggest she is a victim of domestic violence.

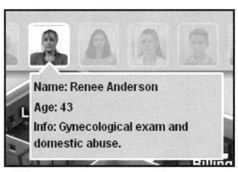

Name: Renee Anderson
Age: 43
Info: Gynecological exam and domestic abuse.

7. **Teresa Hernandez (age 16)**—Teresa is a minor patient who is unaccompanied by a parent for her appointment. She is seeking contraceptive counseling and STD testing.

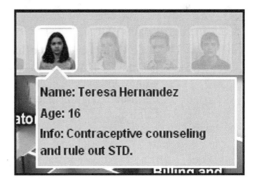

Name: Teresa Hernandez
Age: 16
Info: Contraceptive counseling and rule out STD.

8. **Louise Parlet (age 24)**—Ms. Parlet is an established patient being seen for a pregnancy test and examination. She will also need to be referred to an OB/GYN specialist.

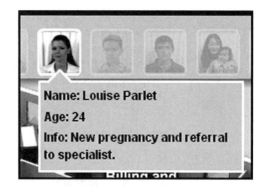

9. **Tristan Tsosie (age 8)**—A minor patient accompanied by his older sister and younger brother, Tristan is having a splint and sutures removed from his injured right arm.

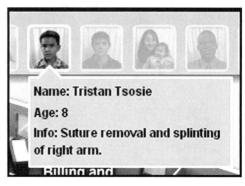

10. **Jose Imero (age 16)**—Jose is a minor patient who is scheduled for an emergency appointment to have the laceration on his foot sutured.

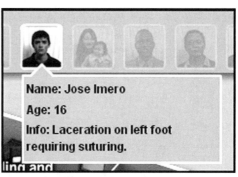

11. **Jade Wong (age 7 months)**—Jade and her parents are new patients to Mountain View Clinic. Jade needs a checkup and updates to her immunizations. Her mother does not speak English.

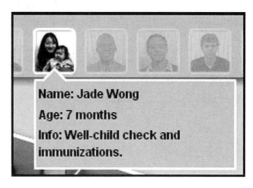

12. **John R. Simmons (age 43)**—Dr. Simmons is a new patient with a history of high blood pressure and recent episodes of blood in his urine.

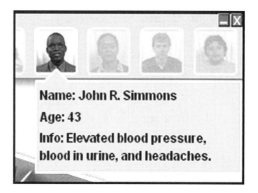

13. **Hu Huang (age 67)**—Mr. Huang developed a severe cough and fever after returning from a recent trip to Asia.

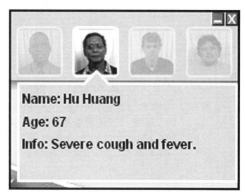

14. **Kevin McKinzie (age 18)**—Mr. McKinzie has made an appointment because of his nausea and vomiting. He is insured through the restaurant where he works.

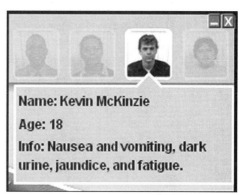

15. **Jesus Santo (age 32)**—Mr. Santo has been brought to the office as a walk-in appointment by his employer for leg pain and a fever. He has no insurance or identification, but his employer has offered to pay for the visit.

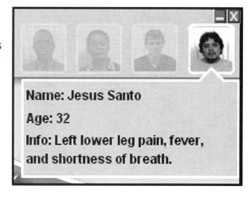

■ BASIC NAVIGATION

HOW TO SELECT A PATIENT

The list of patients is located across the top of the office map screen. Pointing your cursor at the various patients will highlight their photo and reveal their name, age, and medical problem (see examples in the photos on the previous pages). When you click on the patient you wish to review, a larger photo and description will appear in the lower left corner of the screen.

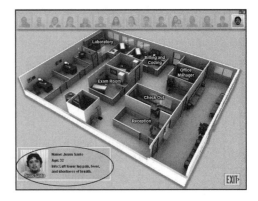

Note: You **must** select a patient before you are allowed access to the Reception area, Exam Room, Laboratory, Billing and Coding office, or Check Out area. The Office Manager area is the only room you can enter without first selecting a patient.

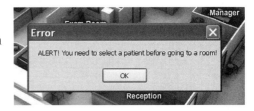

HOW TO SELECT A ROOM

After selecting a patient, use your cursor to highlight the room you want to enter. The active room will be shaded blue on the map. Click to enter the room.

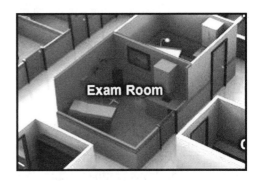

HOW TO LEAVE A ROOM

When you are finished working in a room, you can leave by clicking the exit arrow found at the bottom right corner of the screen.

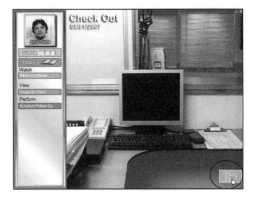

Leaving a room will automatically take you to the Summary Menu.

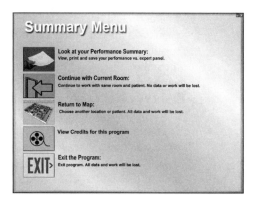

From the Summary Menu, you can choose to:

- **Look at Your Performance Summary**

  In each room there are interactive wizards or tasks that can be completed. The Performance Summary lets you compare your answers with those of the experts.

- **Continue with Current Room**

  This takes you back to the last room in which you worked. This option is not available if you have already reviewed your Performance Summary.

- **Return to Map**

  This reopens the office map for you to select another room and/or another patient.

- **View Credits for This Program**

  This provides a complete listing of software developers, publisher, and authors.

- **Exit the Program**

  This closes the *Virtual Medical Office* software. You will need to sign in again before you can use the program.

HOW TO USE THE PERFORMANCE SUMMARY

If you completed any of the interactive wizards in a room, you can compare your answers with those of the experts by accessing your Performance Summary. The Performance Summary is not a grading tool, although it is valuable for self-assessment and review.

From the Summary Menu, click on **Look at Your Performance Summary**.

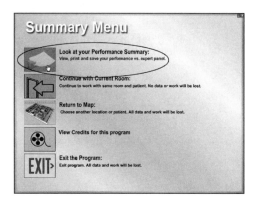

The complete list of tasks associated with the active room will appear with two columns showing the results of your choices. Your answers will appear in the column labeled **Your Performance**, and the answers chosen by the expert will appear in the **Expert's Performance** column. A check mark in the same box in both columns indicates that your answer matched the expert's answer. The Performance Summary can be saved to your computer or disk by clicking on the disk icon at the upper right side of the screen. The saved file can be printed or emailed to your instructor. A hard copy can also be printed without saving by clicking on the printer icon at the upper right corner of the screen.

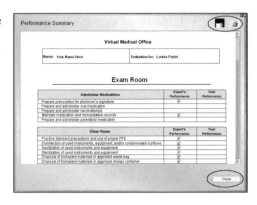

■ ROOM DESCRIPTIONS

Each room can be entered at any time in any order. You can follow a patient's visit from Reception to Check Out, or you can choose to observe each patient at any point in their care. Below is a description of the information and activities that can be found in various rooms.

ALL ROOMS

- In all rooms you can access the patient's medical record and the office Policy Manual.

- In all rooms in which there are interactive tasks to be completed, you can select tasks or features from the menu on the left of the screen, as shown on this sample of the menu in the Reception area.

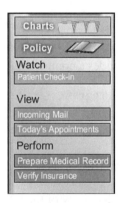

- As an alternative to using the menu, you can click on the corresponding items in the photo of the room. As you move your cursor over each item connected to one of the tasks on the menu, it will highlight and become active.

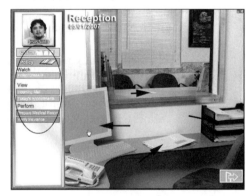

RECEPTION

In the Reception area, you can choose:

- **Charts**—Look at the patient's chart. *Note:* For new patients, there will be no information available in the chart at this time, although you do have the option of assembling a new medical record.
- **Policy**—Open the office Policy Manual and review the established administrative, clinical, and laboratory policies for Mountain View Clinic. Within the Policy Manual you will also find the Coding and Billing Manual.
- **Watch**—Watch a video of the patient's arrival. Each patient is shown checking in at the front desk so that you can observe the procedures typically performed by the receptionist and consider some of the various problems that might arise.
- **Incoming Mail**—Look at the incoming mail for the day. Mountain View Clinic has received a wide range of correspondence that must be read and responded to accordingly.
- **Today's Appointments**—Review the appointment schedule for the day. You can check the schedule to find out what time patients are supposed to arrive, the reason for their visit, and how much time the physician will need for the examination.
- **Prepare Medical Record**—Practice preparing the medical record. This interactive feature allows you to build a medical record for a new patient or update information for an established patient.
- **Verify Insurance**—Verify a patient's insurance. Also interactive, this feature allows you to ask patients about the status of their insurance and to view their insurance cards.

EXAM ROOM

- **Charts** and **Policy**—Access the patient's chart and the office Policy Manual.
- **Watch**—View video clips of different parts of the patient's examination. Observe the actions of the medical assistants in the videos and critique the competencies demonstrated.
- **Exam Notes**—Review the physician's documented findings for the current visit. These notes are added to the full Progress Notes in the patient's chart as the patient continues on to Check Out.
- **Perform**—Perform multiple tasks that are required of a clinical medical assistant, such as preparing the room for the examination, taking vital signs and patient history, and properly positioning the patient for an examination.

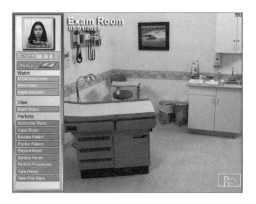

LABORATORY

- **Charts** and **Policy**—Access the patient's chart and the office Policy Manual.
- **View: Logs**—View the laboratory's log of specimens sent out for testing. Opportunities to practice filling out laboratory logs are included in the workbook exercises.
- **Perform**—Perform specific tasks as needed in the laboratory, such as collecting and testing specimens. These interactive wizards walk you through the steps for collecting and testing specimens ordered by the physician as part of the patient's examination. The Progress Notes are available throughout so that you can review the physician's directions.

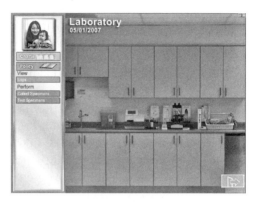

CHECK OUT

- **Charts** and **Policy**—Access the patient's chart and the office Policy Manual.
- **Watch**—Watch a video clip of the patient checking out of the office at the end of the visit. Observe the administrative medical assistants as they schedule follow-up appointments, accept payments, and manage the various duties and problems that may arise.
- **View**—Look at the Encounter Form completed for each patient and verify that the form is filled out correctly and completely.
- **Perform**—Certain patients will require a return visit to the office. Schedule their follow-up appointments as needed. Opportunities to work with the appointment book and additional scheduling tasks are included in the study guide.

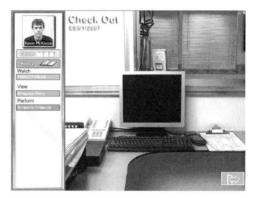

BILLING AND CODING

- **View: Aging Report**—Review the outstanding balances on various patient accounts and assess when to implement different collection techniques.
- **View: Encounter Form**—Review the patient's Encounter Form and determine whether the proper procedures were followed to ensure accurate billing and coding.
- **View: Fee Schedule**—Review the office's fee schedule to calculate the proper charges for the patient's visit.

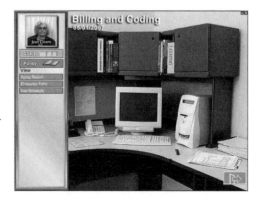

OFFICE MANAGER

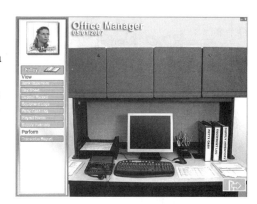

- **Policy**—View the office Policy Manual. Note that patient charts are not available from the manager's office, and there is no need to select a patient to enter the Office Manager area.
- **View**—A variety of financial and administrative documents are available for viewing in the manager's office. Banking deposits and payments can be tracked through these documents, and opportunities to practice managing office finances are included in the study guide.
- **Perform: Transcribe Report**—A recorded medical report is included for transcription practice with full player controls.

■ EMBEDDED ERRORS

The individual lessons and patient scenarios associated with the *Virtual Medical Office* program were designed to stimulate critical thinking and analytical skills and to help develop the competencies on which you will be tested on as part of your course work. Thus deliberate errors have been embedded into each of the 15 patient scenarios and in the Billing and Coding and Office Manager activities. Many of the exercises in the study guide draw attention to these errors so that you can work through how and why a correction needs to be made. Other errors have not been specifically addressed, and you may discover them as you work through the various rooms and tasks. Instructors and students alike are encouraged to use any errors they find to further develop the essential critical thinking and decision-making skills needed for the clinical office.

The following icons are used throughout the study guide to help you quickly identify particular activities and assignments:

 Reading Assignment—tells you which textbook chapter(s) you should read before starting each lesson

 Writing Activity—certain activities focus on written responses such as filling out forms or completing documentation

 Online Activity—marks the beginning of an activity that uses the *Virtual Medical Office* simulation software

 Online Instructions—indicates the steps to follow as you navigate through the software

 Reference—indicates questions and activities that require you to consult your textbook

 Time—indicates the approximate amount of time needed to complete the exercise

Performing Other Professional Duties

/OʒD **Reading Assignment:** Chapter 3—The Medical Assisting Profession
Chapter 4—Professional Behavior in the Workplace
Chapter 5—Interpersonal Skills and Human Behavior

Patient: Rhea Davison

Note: The first exercise does not involve Rhea Davison, but you have to choose a patient to access the clinic rooms.

Learning Objectives:

- Prepare the documentation for possible termination of the patient.
- Describe the necessary documentation of licensure and accreditation.
- Recognize the need for confidentiality and HIPAA regulations.
- Prepare a travel itinerary for a physician who will be speaking at the national AAMA conference.
- Locate resources and information for the employer.
- Describe the need for and the maintenance of liability coverage.

Overview:

In this lesson you will prepare documentation needed for assisting the physician in various areas related to office policies and the physician's professional needs. The ethical and legal aspects of confidentiality are addressed, as well as how to deal with patients who habitually cancel appointments. The Internet will be used to research travel arrangements for a conference one of the physicians needs to attend. Finally, the importance of maintaining liability insurance will be discussed.

Exercise 1

Online Activity—Recognizing the Need for Patient Termination

 45 minutes

- Sign in to Mountain View Clinic.
- Select **Rhea Davison** from the patient list and click on **Reception** to be able to access the schedule.

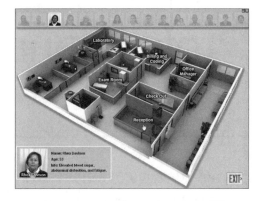

- At the Reception desk, click on **Today's Appointments** to review the day's schedule. You will need to scroll down the appointment book with your mouse to see both the morning and afternoon schedules.

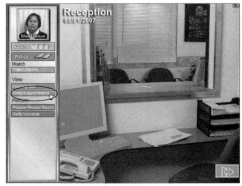

1. Who is the patient who has canceled an appointment, and what was the patient's chief complaint?

Look at your office Policy Manual regarding canceled appointments by following these steps.

- Click **Finish** to close the appointment book and return to the Reception desk. Click on **Policy** to open the office Policy Manual.
- Type "cancel" in the search bar and click the magnifying glass once to read the office policy regarding canceled appointments.

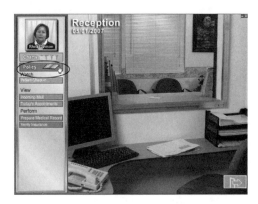

- Click **Close Manual** to return to the Reception desk.

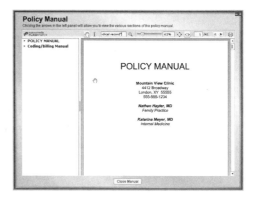

2. What is the role of the medical assistant in providing information about cancellations to the physician?

3. According to the Policy Manual, what is the next step to be taken with this patient who has canceled his last three appointments? Explain your answer.

Exercise 2

Writing Activity

15 minutes

1. Below, compose a letter to the patient you identified in question 1. In the letter, describe the reason for possible termination and the necessary steps needed to remain a patient of Dr. Meyer. The letter should include all of the reasons for possible termination and the need for the patient to keep appointments as made. The letter can also state that Dr. Meyer is concerned about continuity of care and the need for patient safety through this continuity of care.

Mountain View Clinic

4412 Broadway / London, XY 55555 / Phone: (555) 555-1234 / Fax: (555) 555-1239

Nathan Hayler, MD - Family Practice / Katarina Meyer, MD - Internal Medicine

2. Why does the letter need to be sent by certified mail?

Thought Question

3. If a decision is made to terminate a patient, how much time must be allowed between notification and the termination?

• Remain in the Reception area with Rhea Davison and continue to the next exercise.

Exercise 3

Online Activity—Maintaining Licensure and Credentials

 15 minutes

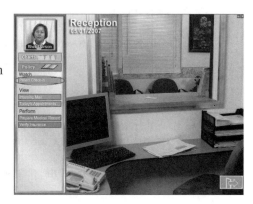

• At the Reception desk with Rhea Davison, click on **Patient Check-In** to view the video. (*Note:* If you have exited the program, sign in again to Mountain View Clinic, select Rhea Davison from the patient list, go to the Reception area, and view the video.)

• At the end of the video, click **Close**.

In the video, the medical assistant discusses the CMA(AAMA) credential. However, the RMA is another credential that is recognized on a national level. *Note:* The CMA credential must now be written as CMA(AAMA) to be distinguished from other CMA credentials that are not Certified Medical Assisting Credentials.

1. Look up the CMA(AAMA) and RMA credentials and name the organizations that award these credentials.

2. Research your state to see if there are any state or regional examinations or credentials awarded by area or region.

3. On arrival this morning, Dr. Meyer states that you need to check on the status of her renewed medical license because it has not arrived. She reminds you that her current license expires on June 1. Go to the Internet and find the name and address of the medical examining board for the state in which you live. Also find the time limit for medical licensure and any necessary components for renewal of the license. Print your findings for your instructor.

➔ • Remain in the Reception area and continue to the next exercise.

Exercise 4

 Online Activity—Maintaining Confidentiality and Explaining Office Policy to the Patient

 40 minutes

- This exercise continues with questions regarding the video of Rhea Davison's check-in. If you need to review the video again, click on **Patient Check-In** at the Reception desk. (*Note:* If you have exited the program, sign in again to Mountain View Clinic, select Rhea Davison from the patient list, go to the Reception area, and view the video again if necessary.)

1. Ms. Davison is an established patient. Did Kristin handle Ms. Davison's late arrival in a professional manner? Explain your answer.

2. Would you have expected Ms. Davison to be upset if her appointment had to be rescheduled?

3. What was your feeling about Kristin and the issue of confidentiality just before the arrival of the office manager?

4. The office manager appeared to be upset with Ms. Davison, but do you think she was more upset with Ms. Davison or with her employee Kristin?

5. The office manager explained the need to follow HIPAA policy and the need for confidentiality of medical records. How do you feel about the attitude of the office manager while discussing the matter of confidentiality?

6. Why does the office manager need to explain the HIPAA policy in such a specific manner?

Exercise 5

Writing Activity—Obtaining Travel Itineraries and Locating Information for the Physician

90 minutes

1. Prepare and provide a travel itinerary for one of the physicians at Mountain View Clinic, following these steps:

   a. Using the Internet as your tool, make travel arrangements for Dr. Meyer to attend the next American Association of Medical Assistants (AAMA) Conference. Dr. Meyer is scheduled to speak on Saturday afternoon at 4 p.m. and would like to arrive at the airport by noon that day. She plans to spend one night and would like a return flight on Sunday arriving no later than 7 p.m.

   b. Decide on the best flight to meet Dr. Meyer's needs from your site (your geographic location) of practice. Record the fare, times of departure and arrival, and any special identification or security requirements.

   c. Make arrangements for Dr. Meyer at the hotel where the conference is to be held, showing the room fee including taxes. Make a notation of the check-in time and the check-out time at the hotel.

   d. Finally, arrange for land transportation for Dr. Meyer from the airport to the hotel and back to the airport. Some hotels have a complimentary shuttle or can recommend a shuttle company. You can also check the price of renting a car or the approximate cost for taxi service.

2. Travel restrictions and requirements change frequently, particularly for travel outside of the United States. Using the Internet as a resource, locate websites that provide updated information on security, restrictions, and requirements for travelers.

3. Dr. Meyer is scheduled to present a speech on sleep apnea at the conference. She asks you to consult the Internet and find five links she can use as information resources as she prepares her speech. What did you find?

(1)

(2)

(3)

(4)

(5)

Exercise 6

Writing Activity—Maintaining Liability Insurance

  15 minutes

1. Why is liability insurance important in the medical office?

2. What steps can the medical assistant take to protect patients from injury in the medical office? List five ways the medical assistant can reduce the chance of accidents.

3. Why is it important for the person responsible for liability insurance to keep a "tickler" file of the dates when premiums are due?

4. Can an electronic date reminder such as one on the Outlook Express calendar be utilized for this purpose to ensure that the premium is paid on time?

2

Telephone Techniques

Reading Assignment: Chapter 5—Interpersonal Skills and Human Behavior
- The Process of Communication

Chapter 9—Telephone Techniques

Patients: Louise Parlet, Wilson Metcalf

Learning Objectives:

- Describe how nonverbal and verbal communication skills are apparent when using the telephone.
- Understand the need for ethical and legal behavior on the telephone.
- Identify ways to ensure confidentiality when using the telephone in the medical office.
- Manage telephone calls professionally while handling other administrative duties.

Overview:

In this lesson, the legal and ethical issues related to the use of the telephone will be discussed. Issues of confidentiality when using the phone to make arrangements for transfer of a patient to an inpatient facility will also be covered. Proper telephone techniques are important in setting the mood for the entire office. This lesson is designed to provide basic understanding of these techniques.

Exercise 1

Online Activity—Proper Use of the Telephone in the Medical Office

 40 minutes

- Sign in to Mountain View Clinic.
- From the patient list, select **Louise Parlet**.

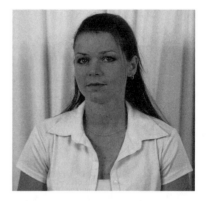

- On the office map, highlight and click on **Reception** to enter the Reception area.

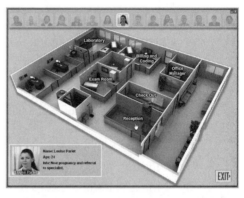

- Under the Watch heading, select **Patient Check-In** to view the video clip.

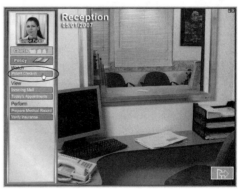

- At the end of the video, click **Close** to return to the Reception desk.

1. As Kristin answers the phone, how does she identify herself? Was her identification a correct procedure? Why or why not?

2. What nonverbal communication does Kristin convey when she answers the phone?

3. Kristin did not close the privacy window while talking on the telephone. Was this a break in confidentiality? Why or why not?

4. When should the privacy window be closed when the medical assistant is on the telephone?

5. Kristin stated "Please excuse me" so that she could answer the telephone. When she completed the phone call, she apologized for the interruption. Was this a proper telephone technique? Give a reason for your answer.

6. What was your opinion about the way the sales representative behaved while Ms. Parlet was at the counter?

7. Could Kristin have handled the sales representative's intrusion into their conversation in a more sensitive way from Ms. Parlet's perspective?

8. Assume that Kristin is engaged in a phone call that involves personal information about the medical condition of a patient. How can she determine whether she is communicating with a person to whom she can legally and ethically release the information?

→ • Click the exit arrow to go to the Summary Menu.
   • On the Summary Menu, click **Return to Map**.

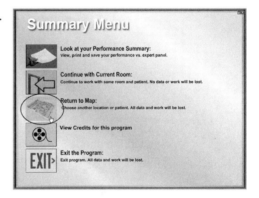

   • From the patient list, select **Wilson Metcalf**.

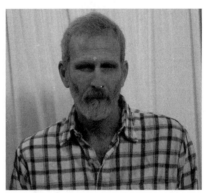

- On the office map, highlight and click on **Check Out**.

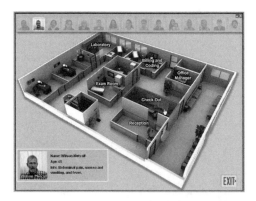

- Under the Watch heading, click on **Patient Check-Out** to view the video clip.

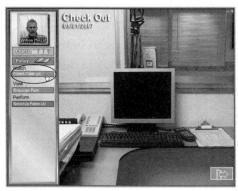

9. How is Mr. Metcalf's confidentiality safeguarded while the medical assistant is on the telephone?

10. How did the medical assistant verify the exact location of the patient transfer so that the orders could be sent as needed?

→ • If you have not already closed the video, click **Close** to return to the Check Out desk.

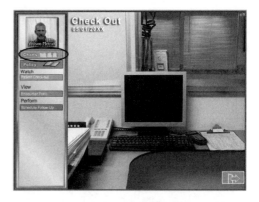

• At the Check Out desk, click on **Charts** and then on the **Patient Information** tab. Select **7-Release of Information Authorization** from the drop-down menu.

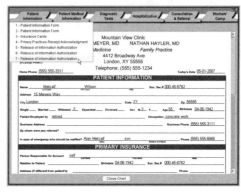

11. Was it permissible for Leah to call Mr. Metcalf's son concerning his transfer to the hospital? Why or why not?

→ • Go to the **Patient Information** tab again, and choose **1-Patient Information Form**. Look for Mr. Metcalf's son's telephone number.

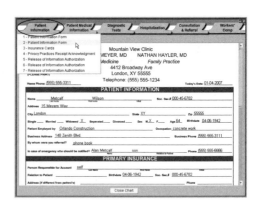

12. What telephone number was given for Mr. Metcalf's son Alan?

13. Would it have been better, in your opinion, to have Mr. Metcalf's son's phone number on the Release of Information Authorization? Why?

Exercise 2

 Writing Activity

 10 minutes

1. List different acceptable ways to introduce yourself if you were working at Mountain View Clinic, keeping in mind the rules for answering the phone that are discussed in your textbook. Practice each way out loud while holding the telephone. Choose which introduction seems most comfortable to you and be prepared to share your personal preference with your classmates.

3

Scheduling and Managing Appointments

Reading Assignment: Chapter 10—Scheduling Appointments

Patient: Janet Jones

Learning Objectives:

- Discuss the rationale for providing space in a day's appointment schedule for emergency appointments.
- Explain the need for a matrix on the appointment schedule.
- Describe the role of the Policy Manual in appointment scheduling.
- Explain the importance of verbal communication concerning appointment delays.
- Apply the skills of scheduling appointments.
- Apply the skills of maintaining the appointment book.
- Identify office policies concerning rescheduling appointments.
- Apply the skills of rescheduling appointments.

Overview:

In this lesson you will schedule and manage appointments using the policies established for this office. The patient, Janet Jones, is upset because she has not been seen immediately. You will discuss the proper way to deal with such a situation. After today's appointment, Janet Jones will need to come back for a follow-up appointment. You will schedule this appointment for her at the appropriate time.

Exercise 1

 Online Activity—Using a Specific Daily Appointment Schedule

25 minutes

- Sign in to Mountain View Clinic
- From the patient list, select **Janet Jones**.

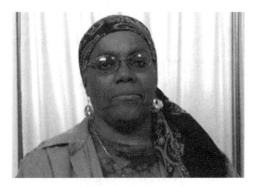

- On the office map, highlight and click on **Reception**.

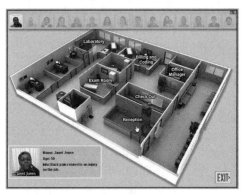

- At the Reception desk, click **Today's Appointments** (under the View heading) to open the appointment book. Review the scheduled appointments, noting the time of Janet Jones' appointment. You will need to scroll down the appointment book to see the entire day.

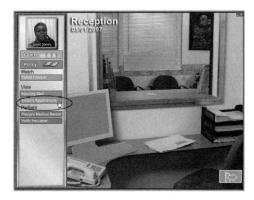

- Click **Finish** to close the appointment book and return to the Reception desk.

1. According to the appointment schedule, what time is Janet Jones' appointment?

2. If Janet Jones signed in at 1:30 p.m., would she have been on time for her appointment? Explain your answer.

• Under the Watch heading, click **Patient Check-In** and watch the video.
• Click **Close** at the end of the video to return to the Reception desk.

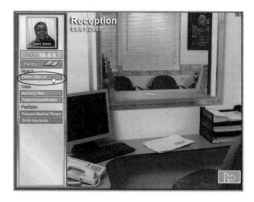

3. Janet Jones is upset when she arrives at the counter. How does Kristin handle the patient in a professional way through verbal and nonverbal communication?

4. Assuming that Ms. Jones checked in at 1:30 p.m., what would have been an appropriate statement for the receptionist to make as the patient checked in to prevent her from becoming so upset?

 • At the Reception desk, click on **Policy** to open the office Policy Manual.

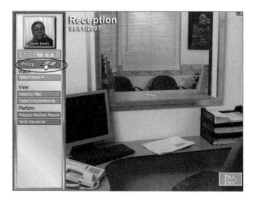

• Type "appointment scheduling" in the search bar and click once on the magnifying glass.

• Read the section of the Policy Manual on scheduling appointments and use this as a tool for answering the questions and scheduling the patient appointments.

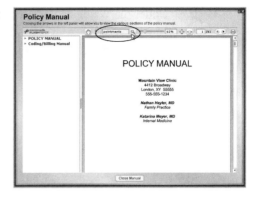

5. How much time is needed for an appointment during which a history and physical examination must be completed for a new patient?

6. Why is it necessary to set up a matrix before making appointments?

7. What buffer times are available for emergency appointments, and why is it important to have this time available?

8. According to the office Policy Manual, what would have been appropriate concerning rescheduling this patient's appointment?

9. Why is it important to identify workers' compensation appointments at the time of scheduling rather than at the time of the appointment?

10. Is the patient's time just as valuable as the physician's time?

- Click **Close Manual** to return to the Reception desk.

- Leave **Reception** by clicking the exit arrow at the lower right corner of the screen.

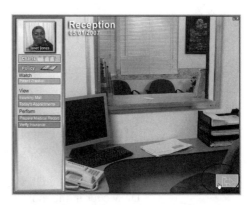

- At the Summary Menu, select **Return to Map** and continue to the next exercise.

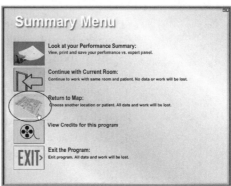

Exercise 2

Writing Activity—Adding Appointments to a Schedule

20 minutes

At the end of the day on April 31, a list of patients needing appointments on May 1 was shown to Dr. Hayler and Dr. Meyer. Both physicians stated that because few patients were currently in the hospital, they would be able to see patients in the clinic earlier than usual the next morning. Dr. Hayler and Dr. Meyer will begin seeing patients at 8:15 a.m. The staff has been informed of the early start. The white areas of the appointment book indicate buffer times for adding patients who need to see the doctor today or for those patients with emergent needs. You may choose a patient, go to the Reception desk, open the Policy Manual, and type "appointment scheduling" in the search bar to review the length of time you will need to block off for each appointment.

1. a. Insert the following appointments for Dr. Hayler into the morning schedule on the next page.

    (1) Robert Leuker is a patient who has not been to the clinic in 5 years and wants to be seen for a lump in his arm. He has a past history of cancer and needs to be seen ASAP. He should be seen first in the morning so that he can be referred as necessary. He is insured through BlueCross/BlueShield (BC/BS). His phone number is (555) 555-8890.

    (2) Lindsey Repp needs a follow-up appointment for an earache and recurrent fever. She is insured through Central Health HMO and can be double-booked at the end of the appointment for Louise Parlet. Her telephone number is (555) 555-9004.

    (3) John Price, who needs a follow-up appointment for his blood pressure, has Medicare. His blood pressure was low when he took it yesterday, and he feels dizzy. He simply wants Dr. Hayler to reevaluate his medication. He can be seen just before lunch. Mr. Price's phone number is (555) 555-1998.

   b. After completing Dr. Hayler's appointments, add the following appointments for Dr. Meyer in the morning, using the same schedule on the next page.

    (1) Catherine Lake needs a follow-up appointment for pyelonephritis. She forgot to make her follow-up appointment when she was last seen. Ms. Lake is going out of town for 2 weeks and needs to see Dr. Meyer before leaving. Her insurance coverage is through BC/BS. Dr. Meyer will see her at the earliest appointment time. Catherine Lake's phone number is (555) 555-1865.

    (2) Lucille Meryl needs to be seen for a follow-up to a thyroid test. Dr. Meyer wants to see her as a double-booking at the end of the appointment for Rhea Davison. Her insurance is through Drake. Her phone number is (555) 555-3219.

    (3) An established patient, Simon Reed, calls at 11:30 a.m. to tell you that he has some chest pain, and even though he has an appointment for tomorrow, he does not think he should wait. Mr. Reed has experienced a heart attack in the past. When you discuss this with Dr. Meyer, she tells you to phone 911 while keeping the patient on the line. She also says that she will go to the hospital to see Mr. Reed once he is in the Emergency Department. What notation should you make on the schedule?

5/1/2007	Dr. Hayler			Dr. Meyer	
	Patient Name	Insurance		Patient Name	Insurance
8:00 AM	(Hospital rounds) Joe Smitty - Chem 12, CBC Marsha Brady - Fasting BS			(Hospital rounds)	
8:15 AM	(Hospital rounds)			(Hospital rounds) Joanne Crosby, PT, PTT (555) 555-1865	
8:30 AM	Louise Parlet, Est. Pt. New Pregnancy/Pelvic (555) 555-3214	Teachers		Rhea Davison, Est. Pt. Elevated BS, abdominal distention, pelvic (555) 555-5656	None
8:45 AM					
9:00 AM					
9:15 AM					
9:30 AM				Hu Huang, Est. Pt. Severe cough, fever (555) 555-1454	Medicare
9:45 AM	Jade Wong, NP 7 mos well child checkup / immunization (555) 555-3345	Central Health HMO			
10:00 AM				~~Chris O'Neil back pain~~ (pt. cancelled - resched 5/7) Jesus Santo, Walk-in Leg pain, SOB	None
10:15 AM					
10:30 AM				Jean Deere, Est. Pt. Memory loss, ear pain (555) 555-6361	Medicare
10:45 AM	Tristan Tsosie, Est. Pt. Suture Removal (555) 555-1515	Blue Cross / Blue Shield			
11:00 AM					
11:15 AM				Wilson Metcalf, Est. Pt. N/V, abdominal pain, difficulty urinating - (555) 555-3311	Medicare
11:30 AM	LUNCH				
11:45 AM					
12:00 PM					
12:15 PM	Renee Anderson, NP Annual GYN Exam (555) 555-3331	Blue Cross / Blue Shield			

2. You must now call John Price to inform him that Dr. Hayler will see him just before lunch. Write the information below that Mr. Price will need to be told. Why did Dr. Hayler need to be contacted before making the appointment for Mr. Price?

3. You must also call Lucille Meryl to inform her that Dr. Meyer wants to see her about her test results. What information do you need to provide, and how would you answer her when she questions why she needs to be seen so quickly?

Exercise 3

Online Activity—Preparing an Appointment Schedule

 30 minutes

- In this exercise we will continue with Janet Jones' visit. If you are already at the office map, click on **Check Out** to go to the Check Out desk. (*Note:* If you have exited the program, sign in again to Mountain View Clinic, select Janet Jones, and go to the Check Out desk.)
- At the Check Out desk, click **Encounter Form** under the View heading.

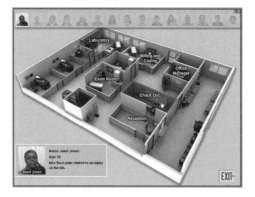

1. At what date should Janet Jones return to the clinic for a follow-up appointment?

2. How much time should be allotted to the follow-up appointment for Ms. Jones?

- Click **Finish** to return to Check Out.
- Click **Patient Check Out** under the Watch heading.

3. At what time of day was Ms. Jones follow-up appointment made?

Complete the following activities using the appointment sheets on the next two pages.

(1) Set up the appointment sheet for the date that Janet Jones is to return for her follow-up visit at the same time the medical assistant in the video scheduled her appointment.

(2) Using the information in the Policy Manual, set up the matrix for that day. (*Note:* If you need to review this, return to the Policy Manual, type "hours of operation" in the search bar, and click once on the magnifying glass.)

(3) Add an appointment at 11:00 a.m. for Kay Soto (an established patient) with Dr. Meyer. Ms. Soto has been prescribed a weight loss program and is coming in for a weight check. Her insurance is through Metro HMO. Ms. Soto's phone number is (555) 555-0954.

(4) George Smith, age 15, is to be seen by Dr. Hayler for a football injury the night before. He has State Agricultural Insurance and is an existing patient. George needs to be seen as early as possible so that he can go to school. Mr. Smith's phone number is (555) 555-8778.

(5) Callie Agree, a new patient, is to be seen for a possible sinus infection. She has Medicare and will be accompanied by her daughter. The daughter prefers to see Dr. Meyer in the midmorning so that her mother will have time to dress. Ms. Agree's phone number is (555) 555-3452.

(6) Sophie Coats, age 6 months, is an established patient who will be seen by Dr. Hayler for a well-baby visit. She is due to have immunizations at this visit. Her mother prefers to have an appointment as early in the morning as possible. Sophie is covered by her father's insurance with Banker's Health. Ms. Coats' phone number is (555) 554-0090.

(7) Mamie Mack, age 18, is an established patient who needs a physical examination for college. She prefers to be seen by Dr. Hayler. Either late morning or early afternoon is better for her since she is still in school. She is covered through George Allen Insurance at her mother's place of employment. Ms. Mack's phone number is (555) 554-8745.

(8) Kay Soto calls to cancel her appointment for the day because she has to leave town to take care of her ill mother. She does not want to reschedule at this time.

(9) Dr. Hayler will need to leave at 11:15 a.m. for a dental appointment but will be back in the afternoon. Mark this on the appointment sheet.

(10) Dr. Meyer is scheduled to be off the afternoon of this day. Mark this on the appointment sheet.

4.

/ /2007	Dr. Hayler		Dr. Meyer	
Time	Patient Name	Insurance	Patient Name	Insurance
8:00 AM				
8:15 AM				
8:30 AM				
8:45 AM				
9:00 AM				
9:15 AM				
9:30 AM				
9:45 AM				
10:00 AM				
10:15 AM				
10:30 AM				
10:45 AM				
11:00 AM				
11:15 AM				
11:30 AM				
11:45 AM				
12:00 PM				
12:15 PM				

5.

/ /2007	Dr. Hayler			Dr. Meyer		
Time	Patient Name		Insurance	Patient Name		Insurance
12:30 PM						
12:45 PM						
1:00 PM						
1:15 PM						
1:30 PM						
1:45 PM						
2:00 PM						
2:15 PM						
2:30 PM						
2:45 PM						
3:00 PM						
3:15 PM						
3:30 PM						
3:45 PM						
4:00 PM						
4:15 PM						
4:30 PM						
4:45 PM						
5:00 PM						

6. Which is the necessary procedure for canceling Kay Soto's appointment?
   a. Erase the canceled appointment and tell Ms. Soto that there will be a charge because she did not give 24 hours notice.
   b. Cross out the appointment (using the office-preferred writing implement) and record the cancellation in the patient medical record.
   c. Report the cancellation to Dr. Meyer.
   d. Tell her that she must reschedule this appointment today for continued medical care.

LESSON 4

Scheduling Admissions and Procedures

Reading Assignment: Chapter 10—Scheduling Appointments
- Scheduling Other Types of Appointments

Chapter 14—The Paper Medical Record
- Releasing Medical Record Information

Patients: Wilson Metcalf, Shaunti Begay

Learning Objectives:

- Recognize the patient information that needs to be sent to a medical facility if your office is making a referral.
- Check the patient's records to verify who is authorized by the patient to receive information regarding the patient.
- Use the Policy Manual to determine the responsibility of the medical assistant in making arrangements for inpatient admissions and referrals to other physicians.
- Explain why it is important to arrange outpatient appointments at a time convenient for the patient.
- Recognize confidentiality issues that must be followed when making arrangements to transfer a patient to a hospital.

Overview:

In this lesson you will make the necessary arrangements for moving Wilson Metcalf from the office to the hospital. You will ensure that his family has been notified of the move. With Shaunti Begay, you will make arrangements for outpatient testing and schedule an office appointment for providing her test results. This patient will also need to see a specialist, so any questions concerning the insurance for these appointments will need to be answered.

49

Exercise 1

Online Activity—Scheduling Inpatient Admissions and Procedures

 30 minutes

- Sign in to Mountain View Clinic.
- From the patient list, select **Wilson Metcalf**.

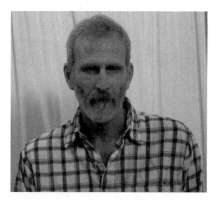

- On the office map, highlight and click on **Check Out**.

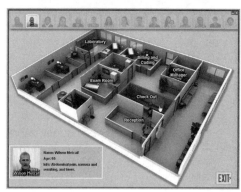

- Click on **Policy** to open the office Policy Manual.
- Type "job description" in the search bar and click once on the magnifying glass.
- Read the section of the Policy Manual concerning the job descriptions for the medical assistants.

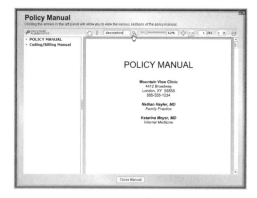

1. According to office policy, which medical assistant has the primary duty of making the arrangements for inpatient admissions and for making referrals to other physicians?

- Click **Close Manual** to return to the Check Out desk.
- Under the Watch heading, select **Patient Check-Out** to view the video. At the end of the video, click **Close**.

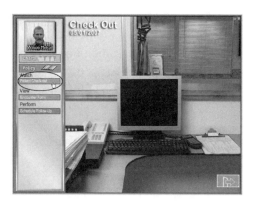

2. Which documents are being copied and sent to the hospital with Mr. Metcalf according to the video? Select all that apply.

_____ Medicare card

_____ Private insurance card

_____ Authorization form

_____ Office registration

_____ Physician's orders

- Click on **Charts** to open Wilson Metcalf's medical record.
- Next, click on the **Patient Information** tab and select **3-Insurance Cards** from the drop-down menu.

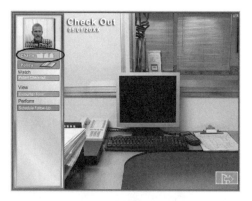

- Click again on the **Patient Information** tab, select **1-Patient Information Form**, and review this form.

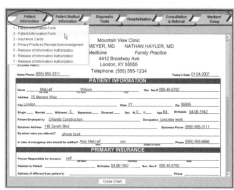

- Once again, click on the **Patient Information** tab. Select **6-Release of Information Authorization Form** from the drop-down menu.
- Note that both the Patient Information Form and the Release of Information Authorization Form are dated 5-1-2007.
- Click **Close Chart** when you have finished reviewing the documents.

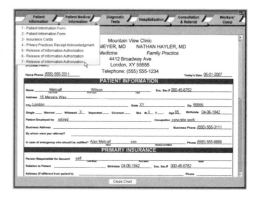

3. Why would it be appropriate to send the office registration and authorization form to the hospital for Wilson Metcalf's admission?

4. Who may receive information concerning Mr. Metcalf's medical condition? Can the entire medical record be released?

5. Did Leah act within the ethical and legal boundaries to release the information she gave to the hospital for Mr. Metcalf? Explain your answer.

6. Why is it important that the window to the waiting room be closed while Leah is making arrangements for Mr. Metcalf to be transferred to the hospital?

Exercise 2

Online Activity—Scheduling Outpatient Admissions and Procedures

 20 minutes

- From the patient list, select **Shaunti Begay**. (*Note:* If you have exited the program, sign in again to Mountain View Clinic and select Shaunti Begay from the patient list.)

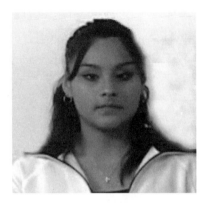

- Highlight and click on **Check Out** on the office map.

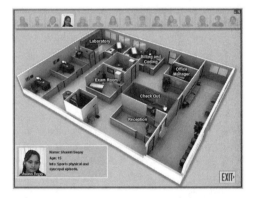

- Select **Charts** to open Shaunti Begay's medical record.

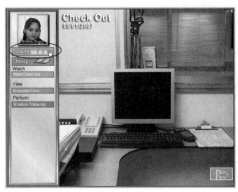

- Under the **Patient Medical Information** tab, select **2-Progress Notes** to read the documentation on the current visit.

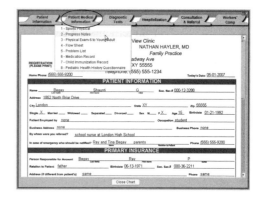

1. What appointments does the medical assistant who is checking patients out need to make?

 - Click **Close Chart**.
- Under the Watch heading, select **Patient Check-Out** to view the video.

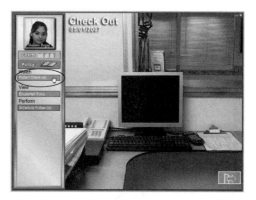

- When you have finished watching the video, click **Close**.

2. Did Leah make sure the referral for outpatient admission and procedures was scheduled at a time convenient for the patient and her family?

3. Why is it important to check that referrals and appointments to specialists are made at a time that is convenient for the patient?

4. Shaunti's father, Mr. Begay, is concerned with the financial aspects of the visit because his insurance is not a provider for this medical office. Leah provided the information about his insurance carrier and the referral. However, she did not provide information that was needed to assist Shaunti in the referral. Can you name two items that were not discussed with Mr. Begay or given to Mr. Begay?

5. Refer back to the Progress Notes and then look at the referral authorization in Shaunti's chart; compare it with the Progress Notes. Did Leah gain approval for all the tests the doctor wants the patient to have?

6. Mr. Begay was concerned about the amount of the bill for Shaunti. Do you think that Leah was professional in her handling of verbal and nonverbal communication in this interaction? In what way, if any, would you have changed what was said or done? Did Leah act in an ethical manner?

- From the Check Out area, click on **Encounter Form** (under the View heading). Review this form.

- Next, under the Perform heading, click on **Schedule Follow-Up**.

- Complete the checklist and click **Finish**.

- Click on the exit arrow at the bottom of the screen to leave the area.

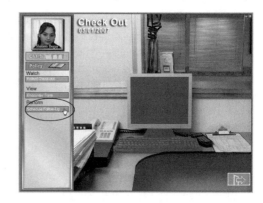

- On the Summary Menu, select **Look at Your Performance Summary** to compare your answers with those of the experts.

- You may save and print the performance summary for your records or to turn in to your instructor.

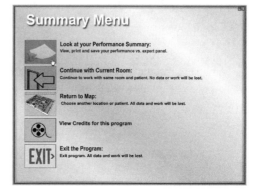

5

Maintaining a Proper Inventory

Reading Assignment: Chapter 12—The Office Environment and Daily Operations
- Supplies and Equipment in the Physician's Office

Patients: None

Learning Objectives:

- Describe the steps necessary for replenishing supplies.
- Discuss how having too many or too few supplies can affect the efficiency of the office.
- Decide which items to reorder and the amount to reorder.
- Explain the necessity of checking equipment for maintenance on a regular basis.
- Discuss the role of the medical assistant in suggesting new equipment for the medical office.
- Describe the proper disposal of controlled substances that are found to be out of date.

Overview:

Ensuring the availability of supplies and equipment when needed is essential to maintaining the efficiency of the medical office practice. The proper inventory of supplies and equipment helps to ensure their availability. In some cases, it is more efficient to order supplies in larger quantities. The medical assistant also has the responsibility of making sure that the equipment ordered is the most currently used in the field. Finally, when medications are found to be out of date, proper disposal is necessary. This lesson will focus on supplies and equipment and their importance to office efficiency.

Exercise 1

Online Activity—Deciding When to Replenish Supplies

30 minutes

- Sign in to Mountain View Clinic.
- On the office map, highlight and click on **Office Manager** to enter the manager's office. (*Note:* You do not need to select a patient for this exercise.)

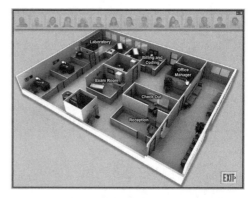

- Click on **Supply Inventory** to view the inventory records.

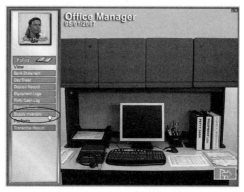

- To view the record for each item in the inventory, click on the corresponding tab headings.

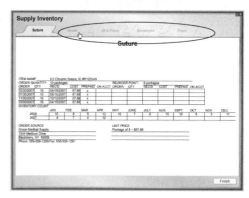

1. What is the reorder point for sutures?

2. Looking at the record from 2006, how many packages of sutures were previously used in May?

→ • Click on the tab heading for **Gauze** to view the inventory record.

3. What is the reorder point for gauze?

4. Looking at the record from 2006, how many bags of gauze were previously used in May?

5. The inventory for gauze is recorded as bags, but gauze can also be ordered by the case. How many bags are in one case?

6. What is the unit price? Does this represent the price per bag or the price per case?

7. What is the discount offered for ordering four or more cases of gauze?

8. After looking at the inventory supply sheet for gauze, should gauze be reordered? If so, why and how much? If not, why not? If you reorder, what will be the net amount of the purchase?

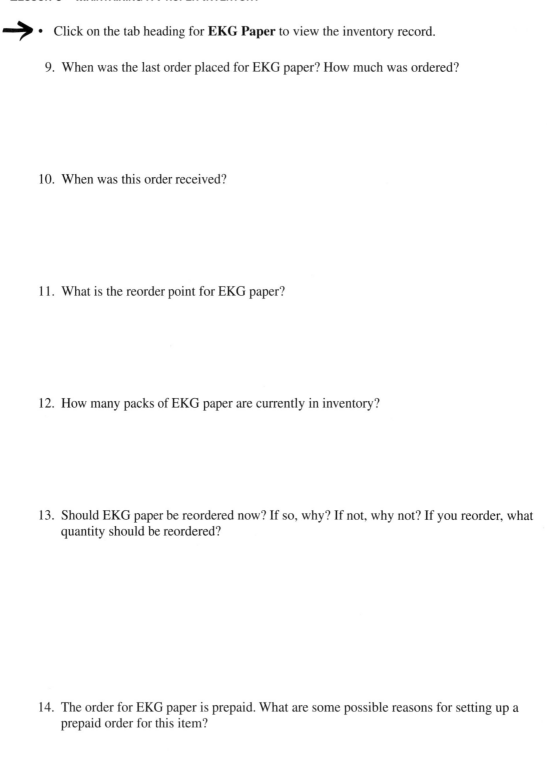 • Click on the tab heading for **EKG Paper** to view the inventory record.

9. When was the last order placed for EKG paper? How much was ordered?

10. When was this order received?

11. What is the reorder point for EKG paper?

12. How many packs of EKG paper are currently in inventory?

13. Should EKG paper be reordered now? If so, why? If not, why not? If you reorder, what quantity should be reordered?

14. The order for EKG paper is prepaid. What are some possible reasons for setting up a prepaid order for this item?

➔ • Click on the tab heading for **Envelopes** to view the inventory record.

15. How often does the office normally order envelopes?

16. On February 28, 2007, the office ordered four more boxes of envelopes. When did this order arrive?

17. Why is there so much time between when the order is placed and when the order is received?

18. From what you see on the inventory form, do the envelopes need to be reordered? How could the office lower the price of the envelopes? Do you see a problem with the reorder point, and does this need to be changed? If the envelopes should be reordered in bulk, what would be the price?

➔ • Click on the tab heading for **Paper** to view the inventory record for copier paper.

19. After examining the inventory supply card for copier paper, what is the cost for three cases?

20. What is the cost for ordering five cases?

21. Below, fill out the purchase order for three cases of copier paper. The shipping fee is $6.00 and the sales tax is 6%.

Office Station

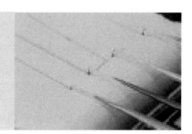

Purchase Order

Bill To:
Mountain View Clinic
4412 Broadway
London, XY 55555

Ship To:
Mountain View Clinic
4412 Broadway
London, XY 55555

Order #:
Date:

Delivery Required By:

Sales Contact	Terms	Tax ID

Item	Quantity	Description	Unit Price	Disc %	Total

Shipping	
Subtotal	
Tax %	
Balance Due	

145 Oceanus Way, St. Pinot, XY 53559
Phone: (123) 456 7890 Fax: (123) 456 7899 CSR@officestation.com

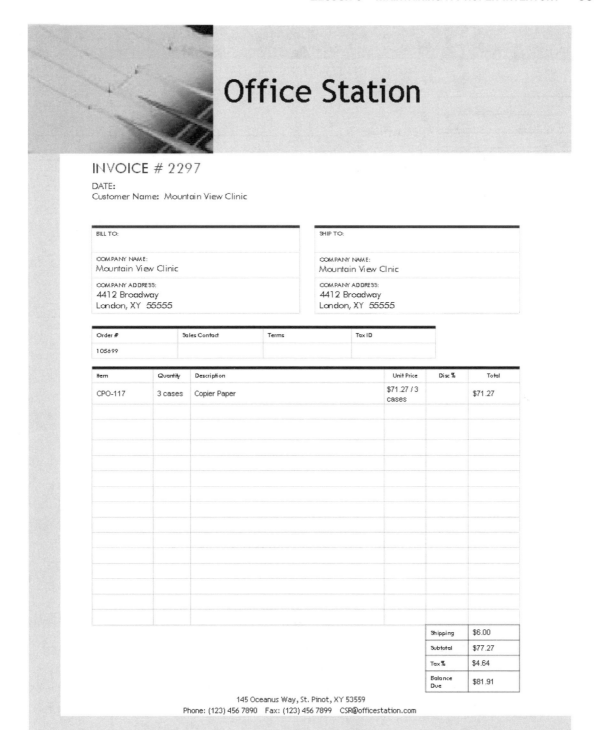

Office Station

INVOICE # 2297

DATE:
Customer Name: Mountain View Clinic

BILL TO:	SHIP TO:
COMPANY NAME: Mountain View Clinic	COMPANY NAME: Mountain View Clinic
COMPANY ADDRESS: 4412 Broadway London, XY 55555	COMPANY ADDRESS: 4412 Broadway London, XY 55555

Order #	Sales Contact	Terms	Tax ID
105699			

Item	Quantity	Description	Unit Price	Disc %	Total
CPO-117	3 cases	Copier Paper	$71.27 / 3 cases		$71.27

Shipping	$6.00
Subtotal	$77.27
Tax %	$4.64
Balance Due	$81.91

145 Oceanus Way, St. Pinot, XY 53559
Phone: (123) 456 7890   Fax: (123) 456 7899   CSR@officestation.com

22. Using the information on the invoice above, complete the check on the next page to pay for the delivered supplies.

| 173980 | | MOUNTAIN VIEW CLINIC | 173980 |

173980

DATE: _____

TO: _____

FOR : _____

ACCOUNT NO. _____

| AMOUNT PAID | $ |

MOUNTAIN VIEW CLINIC
4412 Broadway
London, XY 55555

173980

94-72/1224

Date: _____

Pay to the order of: _____

_____ Dollars $ _____

Clarion National Bank
Member FDIC
90 Grape Vine Road
London, XY 55555-0001

Authorized Signature

|| 005503 || 446782011 || 678800470

23. How should the ordered supplies be handled when they arrive at the office?

Exercise 2

Writing Activity—Properly Disposing Medications

10 minutes

- Sign in to Mountain View Clinic and select any patient from the patient list.
- On the office map, highlight and click on **Reception** to enter the Reception area.
- Click on **Policy** to open the office Policy Manual.
- Type "medications" in the search bar and click once on the magnifying glass.
- Read the section of the Policy Manual concerning the office policy in regard to the disposal of medications.

1. While checking supplies, Cathy notices that some of the nonscheduled medications are out of date. These medications are oral tablets and capsules. What means of disposal is correct for these medications?

2. If part of a schedule II medication ampule has to be disposed of, how many clinical medical assistants need to witness the disposal?

Exercise 3

 Writing Activity—Maintaining Administrative Equipment

10 minutes

1. When filling the copier with paper, Cathy notices that it is time for regular maintenance of the machine and the representative has not been to the office. According to the Policy Manual, the office manager is responsible for maintaining the facilities. What should Cathy's next step be?

2. The toner cartridges are low, and Cathy sees a need for replenishing these. What should she do?

Exercise 4

Writing Activity—Suggestions for Equipment and Supplies

10 minutes

1. Ameeta has observed that not all patients with diabetes are using the same glucose meters at home. The physicians are asking that quality control be checked with patients more often. However, if the office does not have the same glucometers and supplies that some of the patients use at home, it is difficult to provide accurate patient teaching. What steps should Ameeta take to ensure that patient teaching is accurate and helpful for each patient?

2. Leah, as an administrative assistant, has found that the phone line for the fax machine is often busy when a fax needs to be received. Often the person attempting to send the fax has called to complain of the difficulty of getting important information to the physicians. What steps should Leah take to show the need for another fax line for the hospital?

Written Communications

⟋ᴏᴢᴐ **Reading Assignment:** Chapter 13—Written Communication and Mail Processing

Patient: Wilson Metcalf

Learning Objectives:

- Prepare letters in response to the mail received.
- Use correct grammar, spelling, and formatting techniques in letter writing.
- Read mail correspondence correctly.

Overview:

In this lesson you will be asked to respond to incoming mail that includes an NSF check and a letter from a collection agency.

Exercise 1

Online Activity—Reading Mail and Composing a Letter for an NSF Check

 40 minutes

- Sign in to Mountain View Clinic.
- From the patient list, select **Wilson Metcalf**.

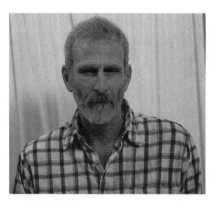

- On the office map, highlight and click on **Reception** to enter the Reception area.

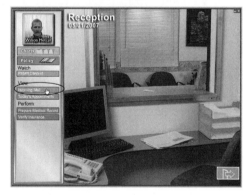

- Under the View heading, select **Incoming Mail** to view the mail received by the clinic.
- Click the numbers to examine and read each piece of mail.

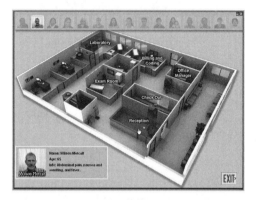

1. Were any payments received in the mail today?

2. List the people from whom payments were received.

3. What is the name of the physician who sent a consultation letter to Dr. Meyer?

4. Who was the letter in reference to?

 • From the list of mail at the top of the screen, click on **7** to view that piece of mail again.
• Leave the Incoming Mail window open as you complete the remaining exercises.

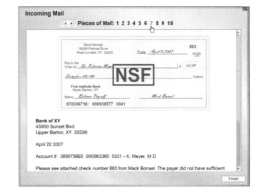

5. On the next page, write your letter to the patient about the NSF check, using an acceptable format. Be sure your message conveys the need to handle this matter within a certain number of days. Also inform the patient that no further checks will be accepted for this patient's medical care at Mountain View Clinic. This should be prepared for a signature by the office manager.

Mountain View Clinic

4412 Broadway / London, XY 55555 / Phone: (555) 555-1234 / Fax (555) 555-1239

Nathan Hayler, MD - Family Practice / Katarina Meyer, MD - Internal Medicine

Exercise 2

Online Activity—Composing a Letter in Response to an Inaccurate Accounts Payable

 30 minutes

- From the list of mail at the top of the screen, click on **10** to read the letter from Summer Oxygen Company.
- Click **Finish** to return to the Reception Desk.

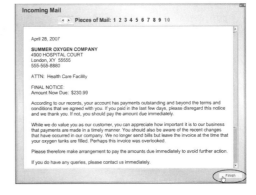

- Click the exit arrow to leave the Reception area.
- On the Summary Menu, click **Return to Map**.

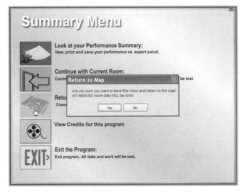

- On the office map, highlight and click on **Office Manager** to enter the manager's office.

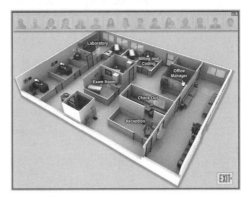

- Under the View heading, click on **Bank Statement** to view the most recent statement from the bank.

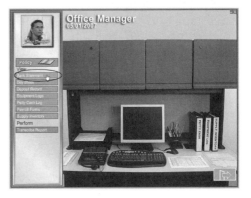

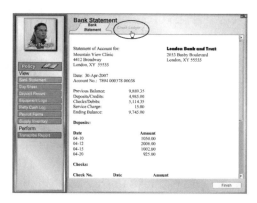

- Select the **Check Ledger** tab to review the most recent checks written by Mountain View Clinic.

1. There was a payment made to Summer Oxygen Company for $230.99.

   a. According to the check ledger, what was the date the payment was made?

   b. What was the check number?

- Click on the **Bank Statement** tab to review the account activity for April 2007.

2. Did check #1230 for $230.99 clear the account, according to the bank statement?

- Click **Finish** to return to the manager's office.

3. Below, compose a letter to the oxygen supply company in response to the claim that the invoice has not been paid. Write your letter using an acceptable format. Be sure your message includes all information needed to clear the accounts payable. This should be prepared for signature by the office manager.

Mountain View Clinic

4412 Broadway / London, XY 55555 / Phone: (555) 555-1234 / Fax (555) 555-1239

Nathan Hayler, MD - Family Practice / Katarina Meyer, MD - Internal Medicine

Organizing a Patient's Medical Record

Reading Assignment: Chapter 14—The Paper Medical Record
- Creating an Efficient Medical Records Management System
- Organization of the Medical Record
- Contents of the Complete Case History
- Making Additions to the Patient Record
- Keeping Records Current

Chapter 15—The Electronic Medical Record
- Executive Order to Promote Interoperability of EMR Systems
- Technological Terms in Health Information

Patients: Renee Anderson, Tristan Tsosie

Learning Objectives:

- Discuss why proper organization of the medical record is essential.
- Identify and describe the forms found in a medical record.
- Apply principles of medical record organization to choose forms that would be needed when preparing a new patient's medical record.
- Determine if forms need to be added to the medical record for an established patient.
- Describe the appropriate care of a damaged medical record.
- Determine the appropriate division of medical records when a new record must be established.
- Understand the difference between the terms Electronic Health Record (EHR), Electronic Medical Record (EMR), and Personal Health Record (PHR).
- Identify the goal of EMR interoperability.

Overview:

In this lesson we will explore the importance of preparing a patient's medical record correctly. Because the medical record is a legal document that shows the chronological care of the patient, this document must be correctly organized to ensure that information can be located as needed. Incorrectly organized charts not only cause frustration, but also decrease the efficiency of the medical practice. In this lesson you will organize a medical record for a new patient. For an established patient, you will ensure that information received from other sources has been properly organized and that the information is readily available when the patient arrives for an appointment. You will also be asked to distinguish between the terms Electronic Medical Records and Electronic Health Records.

Exercise 1

Online Activity—Organizing a Medical Record for a New Patient

 30 minutes

- Sign in to Mountain View Clinic.
- From the patient list, select **Renee Anderson**.

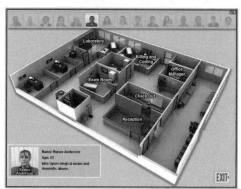

- Highlight and click on **Reception** on the office map.

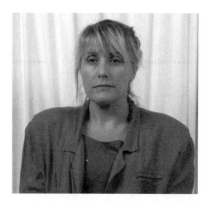

- Click on **Policy** to open the Policy Manual. In the search bar, type "medical record" and click on the magnifying glass to search.

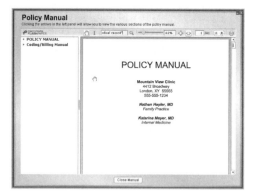

- Scroll up and down to read the duties assigned to the various types of medical assistants in the office.

1. At Mountain View Clinic, the Policy Manual states that the _____ medical assistant is responsible for preparing and organizing the medical record.

2. Why is it important for the administrative medical assistant to provide the necessary forms in a medical record for a new patient?

3. Follow the directions below to assemble a medical record. Your selections will be compared against those of an expert during the Performance Summary.

• When you have finished reading the relevant policy, click on **Close Manual** to return to the Reception desk.

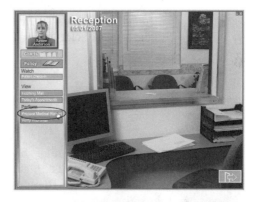

• At the Reception desk, click on **Prepare Medical Record** (under the Perform heading) to begin assembling a chart for Ms. Anderson's visit.

• Next, go to Assemble Medical Record and click on **Perform** to begin selecting the forms necessary for Ms. Anderson's visit.

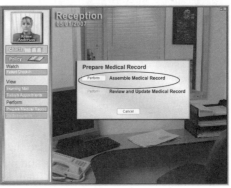

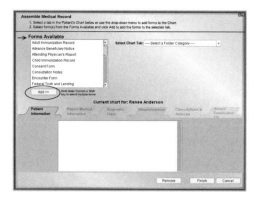

- The Patient Information tab is automatically chosen as the starting point when you access the Assemble Medical Record screen. Under Forms Available, choose the forms that should be filed under the Patient Information tab. Click **Add** to complete your selections. (*Note:* To select multiple consecutive forms, hold down the Shift key while making your selections. To make multiple nonconsecutive selections, hold down the Control [Ctrl] key as you click on your choices.) If you change your mind about a form you have added to a tab, click to highlight the name of the form and then click on **Remove** at the bottom of the screen.

- Make note of which forms you add in the space below.

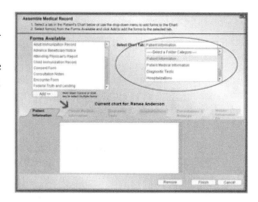

- When you have completed the Patient Information section, continue adding forms to the appropriate tabs in Renee Anderson's medical record. To select a new tab, either click on the tab on the medical record itself or use the drop-down menu to the right of Select Chart Tab.

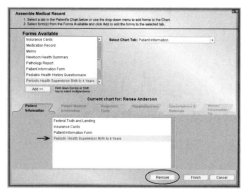

- If you change you mind about a form you have added to a tab, click to highlight the name of the form and then click **Remove** at the bottom of the screen.

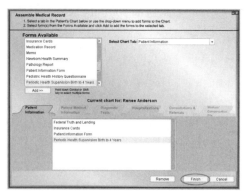

- When you are satisfied that you have selected all the necessary forms and put them in the correct tab sections, click **Finish** to close the medical record.

- Now click on the exit arrow at the bottom of screen to leave the Reception area.

• On the Summary Menu, click on **Look at Your Performance Summary** to compare your answers against those of the experts. How did you do?

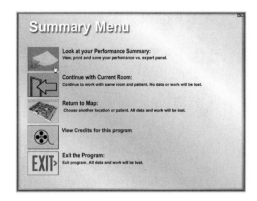

• The icons for saving and printing the Performance Summary are located at the top right corner of the screen. (*Note:* If you do not save your Performance Summary, all data will be lost when you return to the map.)

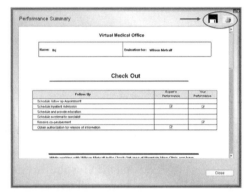

• Click **Close**.
• Click **Return to Map**.

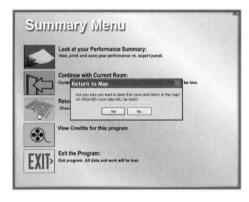

4. The form that contains the patient's demographic information is the

_____.

5. The form in the medical record that contains subjective information about the patient's

illnesses in the past is the _____.

6. The legal document that must be signed to allow information to be used to file insurance is

the _____.

7. The form used at each visit that allows the physician to record findings in the medical

record is the _____.

Exercise 2

Online Activity—Determining Whether to Add Forms to the Medical Record of an Established Patient

 20 minutes

- From the patient list, click on **Tristan Tsosie**. (*Note:* If you have exited the program, sign in again to Mountain View Clinic and select Tristan Tsosie from the patient list.)

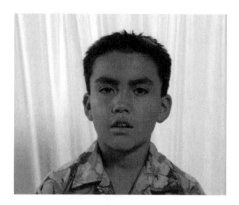

- On the office map, click on **Reception**.
- At the Reception desk, click on **Charts**.
- Click on the **Hospitalization** tab. From the drop-down menu, select **1-ED Record**.
- Read the ED Record to decide what other forms should be available for the physician for this office visit and to determine whether Tristan is following the orders of the physician who saw him in the Emergency Department. Think about which procedures the patient had while at the Emergency Department and which procedure should have a report to be filed in his chart. Then look under the tabs to see if you can find the report that you would also need to have available for the physician.

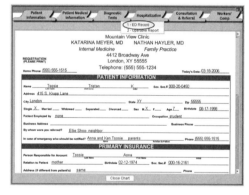

- Click on **Close Chart** to return to the Reception area.
- Under the Perform heading, select **Prepare Medical Record**.
- Click on the **Perform** button next to Review and Update Medical Records.

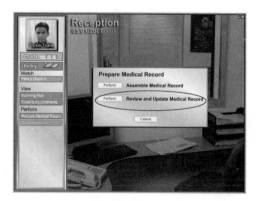

• Check the forms in each chart tab to be sure that the needed information for this visit is located under the correct tab and will be available when the physician needs it. Add any forms that you think are needed for this visit. If you think it is necessary, you may also remove or move any forms within the chart. (*Note:* If you need help with these steps, see the detailed instructions in Exercise 1 of this lesson.)

• When you are done, click **Finish** and then click the exit arrow to leave the Reception area.

• On the Summary Menu, click **Look at Your Performance Summary**.

All of the forms were in the chart that will be needed for Tristan's visit. His ED report and the radiology report were in his health record.

1. Explain the difference between the terms Electronic Medical Record (EMR) and Electronic Health Records (EHR).

2. If the medical office were sharing information with the hospital, would the record be called EMR or EHR?

3. Did the Emergency Department report advise the patient of when (number of days) to follow up with the doctor? Could this omission of information lead to problems with the patient's follow-up care?

4. Was (were) the report(s), other than the ED Record, available in the record?

5. When adding a report to the medical record, the medical assistant should:
   a. be sure the physician has seen the report before filing it.
   b. place the forms in the medical record in chronological order, with the earliest record on top.
   c. always be sure the date of arrival has been stamped on the form.
   d. wait to file the form just before the patient's arrival for an appointment.
   e. do both a and d.

6. When the medical assistant files materials in the medical record of an established patient, the materials should be filed in what order?

7. When accessing Tristan's medical record on arrival, you notice that the forms from the hospital have been torn during transmittal. What steps do you need to take to protect the record from further damage?

8. If a patient's folder is old, torn, or simply worn, what should the medical assistant do?

9. If a chart is overcrowded and a second chart needs to be established, how far back should the records that are moved to the new chart go? How should the record be marked to show that more than one medical record is available?

10. If the medical office is using an EMR that is interoperable with the hospital's EMR, would the physician have been able to access Tristan's records without having a paper copy in the medical record?

11. What is the goal of EMR interoperability?

12. Who manages, shares, and has control of the information in the Personal Health Record (PHR)?

Filing Medical Records

👓 **Reading Assignment:** Chapter 14—The Paper Medical Record
- Creating an Efficient Medical Records Management System
- Filing Procedures
- Filing Methods
- Organization of Files

Chapter 15—The Electronic Medical Record
- Technological Terms in Health Information
- Capabilities of EMR Systems

Patients: All

Learning Objectives:

- Alphabetize patient names for efficiency in filing medical records.
- List the necessary steps needed to prepare a paper medical record for filing.
- Describe the use of color coding to enhance paper medical record systems.
- Identify the filing systems used most frequently in the medical office for patient records.
- Discuss the differences between alphabetic and numeric filing systems.
- Determine which patients are established patients and which are new patients for preparing charts.
- Discuss the means for finding displaced paper medical records.
- Explain the most important function of primary features that EMR software may offer.

Overview:

Proper filing of medical records is essential in providing continuity of care for patients. You will determine if patients are new or established in preparation for filing and you will then alphabetize patients. You will be asked to differentiate between alphabetic and numeric filing systems and identify methods for locating misplaced medical information. One activity will involve answering questions about the different features with which typical EMR software comes.

Exercise 1

Online Activity—Preparing Patient Medical Records for Filing

🕙 50 minutes

- Sign in to Mountain View Clinic.
- One at a time, select each patient from the patient list across the top of the page (moving from left to right) and record his or her name in the table in question 1 below.

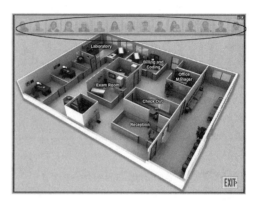

1. Record the names of all of the Mountain View Clinic patients in the first and third columns of the table below. Fill in all of column 1 first; then continue at the top of column 3.

Patient Name	First Date of Service; Last Date of Service	Patient Name	First Date of Service; Last Date of Service

•   Now click again on any patient in the patient list. Then on the office map, click on **Reception**. At the Reception desk, click on **Today's Appointments** to view the day's schedule. Look for each patient's name and note next to his or her name in the table in question 1 whether that patient is a new patient (NP) or an established patient (Est. Pt.) (*Note:* You will return to fill in the remaining columns of the table later in this exercise.)

2. With the schedule of Today's Appointments still open, make a list below of the patients Dr. Hayler is to see in the morning. Place these patients in the correct order for their appointments and note whether the medical record can be pulled from the files of established patients or whether a new record should be prepared.

3. What medical records will need to be pulled from the files for Dr. Meyer's morning patients? Will any of these patients need to have a new record prepared? List these patients and their record needs below (in the order of their appointment times).

•   Click **Finish** to close the appointment book and return to the Reception desk.
•   Click the exit arrow in right lower corner of screen.

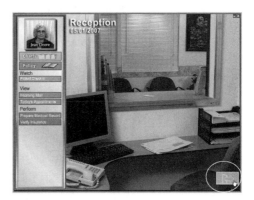

- From the Summary Menu, click on **Return to Map**; then click **Yes** to return to the office map and select another patient.

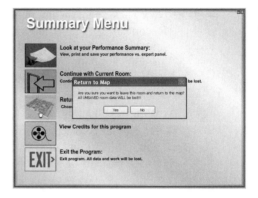

- Beginning with the first patient on the left in the patient list, click on **Reception**. Open the patient's chart, click on the **Patient Medical Information** tab, and select **Progress Notes**. Based on what you find, record the patient's first and last dates of service in columns 2 and 4 in the table in question 1.

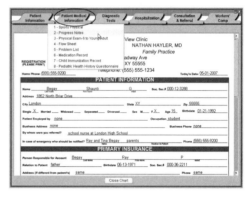

Important: New patients will not have any forms in their chart. Use today's virtual date—5-1-07—as their first date of service; there will be no "last date of service" for new patients.

- When you have recorded the date(s) for the first patient, click **Close Chart**; then click the exit arrow.
- From the Summary Menu, click on **Return to Map**.
- Select your next patient, open the chart, and record the date(s) in the table.
- Continue these steps for each patient until you have completed the table in question 1.

4. Using the table in question 1 as a reference, list the patients' names in alphabetic order in the left column below. In the right column indicate whether the medical records for each patient will be available in the file cabinet of established patients or whether the record will have to be organized and placed in the correct position as a new medical record.

Alphabetic List of Patients	New or Established Record?

5. As you pull the medical records for established patients, you will need to change the year on the medical records for these patients (unless the patient has already been seen in the current year). List the established patients below and indicate what year will need to be relabeled on their medical record (if this applies). Remember, today's virtual date is May 1, 2007.

Name of Established Patient	Year That Will Need to Be Relabeled

6. At the end of the morning, the medical records need to be filed correctly to prevent loss and to ensure proper time management. Below, list in alphabetic order the names of patients who had morning appointments today and whose records will need to be refiled.

Exercise 2

Writing Activity

25 minutes

Answer the following questions regarding paper medical records and capabilities of EMR systems.

1. Which of the following would not be used to help prevent misfiling of medical records?
   a. Colored letter tabs for use with names
   b. Colored tabs for the last year seen in the office
   c. Outguides
   d. Alphabetic tabs in the filing system

2. The two paper filing systems most often used in a medical office are

   _____ and _____ filing.

3. Describe the differences in alphabetic and numeric filing systems.

4. Explain how color-coding enhances paper medical record systems?

5. List the five steps needed to prepare a paper medical record for filing.

   (1)

   (2)

   (3)

   (4)

   (5)

6. What steps can be followed for "finding" a misplaced paper medical record?

7. Explain the primary function of the following features of EMR software systems:

a. Specialty software

b. Appointment scheduler

c. Appointment reminder and confirmation

d. Prescription writer

e. Medical billing systems

f. Charge capture

g. Eligibility verification

h. Referral management

i. Laboratory order integration

j. Patient portal

Insurance Forms and Verification

Reading Assignment: Chapter 18—Basics of Diagnostic Coding
Chapter 19—Basics of Procedural Coding
Chapter 20—Basics of Health Insurance
Chapter 21—The Health Insurance Claim Form

Patients: Shaunti Begay, Louise Parlet, John R. Simmons, Janet Jones, Jose Imero

Learning Objectives:

- Apply managed care policies and procedures to office billing and coding.
- Use third party guidelines for preparing insurance claims and collecting copayments.
- Verify insurance information and initiate a referral for a patient.
- Determine which diagnosis should be coded, and which should not, from patient documentation in the chart.
- Proofread an insurance claim form and identify errors that will affect claims processing.

Overview:

In this lesson you will perform the necessary steps to prepare a clean claim for insurance purposes and collecting copayments that are due to the practice. Completing these steps requires the correct use of managed care policies and procedures and the proper application of the office Policy Manual. A clean claim includes the appropriate diagnostic and procedural codes as well as the proper completion of the insurance claim form. You will proofread an insurance form and compare it with the information in the patient's chart and Encounter Form. You will indicate which boxes need corrections before the claim can be sent to the insurance company.

Exercise 1

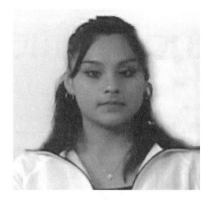

Online Activity—Verifying Insurance for a New Patient

30 minutes

- Sign in to Mountain View Clinic.
- From the patient list, select **Shaunti Begay**.

- On the office map, highlight and click on **Reception**.

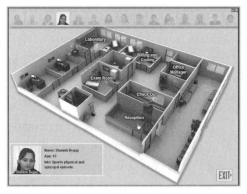

- At the Reception desk, click on **Policy** to open the office Policy Manual.

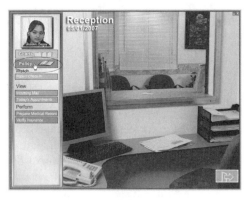

- Type "payment" in the search bar and click the magnifying glass once. This will take you to page 14 of the Policy Manual. Under the Telephone Policies heading, the sixth bullet reminds the medical assistant to inform patients that the copay or their portion of payment is due at the time of service.

- Type "patient insurance policies" in the search bar and click the magnifying glass once. This will take you to page 17 of the Policy Manual. Scroll up to adjust the page and read the policies that apply when patients have insurance coverage that is not accepted by the medical practice.

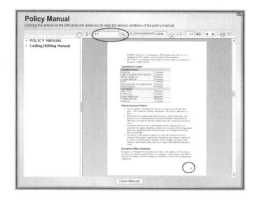

1. According to the Policy Manual, what information should be obtained from the patient when the appointment is made?

2. Why is it important for the medical assistant to verify whether the office is a preferred provider with the patient's insurance at the time the appointment is made?

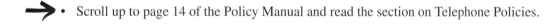

- Scroll up to page 14 of the Policy Manual and read the section on Telephone Policies.

3. What does the Policy Manual state about collecting payments, copays, and percentages of charges for patient visits?

- Click **Close Manual** to return to the Reception desk.
- Click on **Patient Check-In** to view the video of Shaunti's arrival at the clinic.

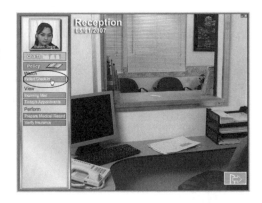

- At the end of the video, click **Close** to return to the Reception desk.
- At the Reception desk, click on **Verify Insurance** to obtain the required information for Shaunti's visit.

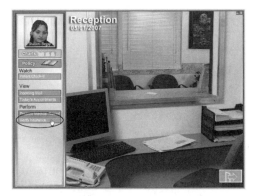

- Select the appropriate question to ask Shaunti regarding her insurance; then click **Insurance Card(s)** to review the insurance cards on the next screen.

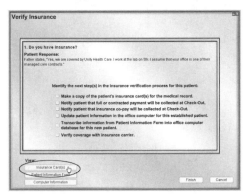

- Click **Finish** to return to the Reception desk.
- Click again on **Policy** to reopen the Policy Manual.
- From the menu on the left side of the screen, click on the arrow next to **Coding/Billing Manual**. The menu will expand. View the additional headings for that section of the Policy Manual.
- Click the arrow next to **Financial Policy** and select **Accepted Insurance Carriers** from the list. You may use the magnifying glass if needed.
- Click **Close Manual** to return to the Reception desk.

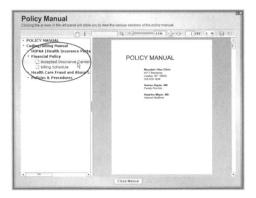

4. Was Kristin correct in stating that Mountain View Clinic was not a participating provider for Shaunti's insurance plan?

5. What did Shaunti's mother say about the information she gave the receptionist regarding their insurance coverage when she made the appointment?

6. What steps should the medical assistant have taken to avoid the confusion that occurred when Shaunti checked in?

→ • Click the exit arrow to leave the Reception desk.
  • From the Summary Menu, select **Return to Map**.

Exercise 2

 Online Activity—Obtaining a Referral for an Established Patient

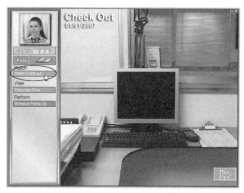 30 minutes

- Select **Louise Parlet** from the patient list. (*Note:* If you have exited the program, sign in again to Mountain View Clinic and select Louise Parlet from the patient list.)

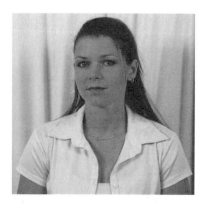

- On the office map, highlight and click on **Check Out**.

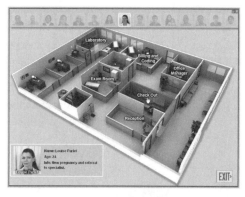

- At the desk, click on **Patient Check-Out** to view the video.

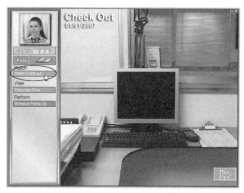

- At the end of the video, click **Close** to return to the desk.

1. Why is it important that the medical assistant assist Ms. Parlet in obtaining approval from her insurance company for the referral to Dr. Lockett?

2. After receiving the precertification verification number, how should the medical assistant handle the verification number?

 • Next, click on **Charts** to open Ms. Parlet's medical record.
 • Under the **Patient Medical Information** tab, select **3-Progress Notes** and read Dr. Hayler's notes regarding the examination.

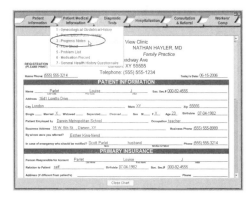

3. What instructions does Dr. Hayler give about the results of the lab work?

Critical Thinking Question

4. Do you think most insurance companies would reimburse a medical provider for a test if the test has already been completed at another facility?

 • Click **Close Chart** to return to the Check Out desk.
 • Click the exit arrow; from the Summary Menu, select **Return to Map**.

Exercise 3

Online Activity—Choosing the Correct Diagnosis to Code for an Office Visit of a New Adult Patient

 30 minutes

- Select **John R. Simmons** from the patient list. (*Note:* If you have exited the program, sign in again to Mountain View Clinic and select John R. Simmons from the patient list.)

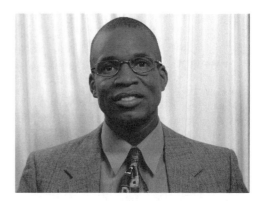

- On the office map, highlight and click on **Billing and Coding**.

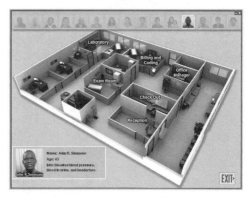

- At the Billing and Coding desk, click on **Encounter Form** to view the diagnostic and procedural information for Dr. Simmons' visit.

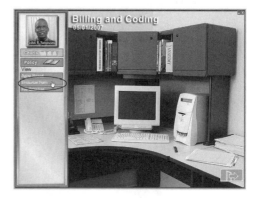

- Your instructor may ask you to use the ICD-10 to choose the correct numeric codes for the diagnoses listed.
- *Important:* Please remember that your codes will be from the ICD-10, not ICD-9, even though the Encounter Form says the clinic is using ICD-9.

1. In the ICD-9 section of the Encounter Form, which diagnoses are checked off for Dr. Simmons' visit?

2. Which of these diagnoses should receive an ICD-9 code? If there are any diagnoses that should not be coded, explain why not.

3. When should the Hemoccult test that the patient will collect at home be billed? Explain your answer.

 • Click **Finish** to close the Encounter Form and return to the Billing and Coding desk.
   • Click on **Charts** to open Dr. Simmons' medical record.
   • Under the **Patient Information** tab, select **5-Insurance Cards** from the drop-down menu.

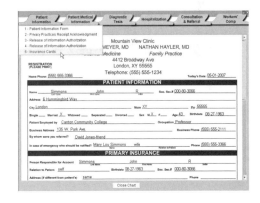

4. What is meant by PCP?

5. What is meant by POS?

6. Using the information on the insurance cards found in the medical record, what is the copay on the patient's insurance? What is the payment rate on the secondary insurance?

7. Look at the back of both of the insurance cards. What do you notice when comparing the cards?

➤ • Click **Close Chart** to return to the Billing and Coding desk.
   • Click the exit arrow; from the Summary Menu, select **Return to Map**.

Exercise 4

Online Activity—Insurance Versus Workers' Compensation Claims

30 minutes

- From the patient list, select **Janet Jones**. (*Note:* If you have exited the program, sign in again to Mountain View Clinic and select Janet Jones from the patient list.)

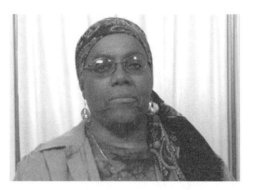

- On the office map, highlight and click on **Billing and Coding**.

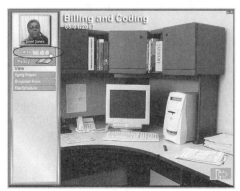

- Click on **Charts** to open Janet Jones' medical record.
- Next, click on the **Patient Information** tab.

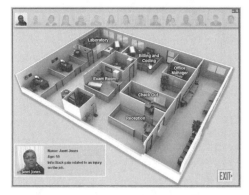

1. You will notice that in Ms. Jones' medical record, there is no information about private insurance coverage. Why is this important for this case?

2. If a patient says that he or she were injured at the workplace or has a work-related illness, what would the medical assistant need to do prior to escorting the patient to the examination room? Refer to the Workers' Compensation section in Chapter 20 of the textbook if you need help locating the answer.

→ • Now click on the tab labeled **Workers' Comp**.

3. What information do you find under this tab in Ms. Jones' medical record?

4. Can you give an example of an injury or a problem for which the insurance company might not pay if the patient had previous problems with the same or a similar diagnosis?

Exercise 5

Other Activity—Proofreading and Critical Thinking Exercise

45 minutes

Jose Imero's insurance claim has been filled out by the medical assistant student. Your responsibility is to review the insurance form and make sure it is correct prior to billing the insurance company. There are several errors on the form. You will use the textbook, the Patient's Information Form, the Insurance Card, the Progress Notes, and the Encounter Form to ensure that everything on the form is correct. Review Chapter 21 in the textbook carefully before you begin this exercise, and use it as a tool as you review the insurance form.

- From the patient list, select **Jose Imero**.
  (*Note:* If you have exited the program, sign in again to Mountain View Clinic and select Jose Imero from the patient list.)

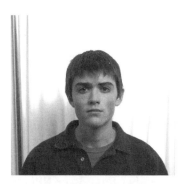

- On the office map, highlight and click on **Billing and Coding**.

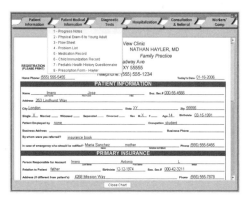

- Click on **Charts** to open Jose Imero's medical record. Then click on the **Patient Information** tab.
- From the drop-down menu, select **1-Patient Information Form** to review the patient's demographic information, which will be used to compare the first portion of the insurance form. When finished, select **2-Insurance Cards** to verify that the insurance identification numbers are correct.
- When you get to box 14 on the insurance claim form, click on the **Patient Medical Information** and choose **1-Progress Notes**. When finished, click **Close Chart**.

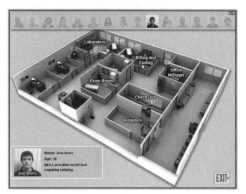

- When you get to box 24 on the insurance claim form, click on **Encounter Form** (under View) in the Billing and Coding office area to see what services the patient received. Click **Finish** when done.
- Select **Fee Schedule** (under View) in the Billing and Coding office area to make sure the insurance form has the correct amount for each service listed. Click **Finish** when done.

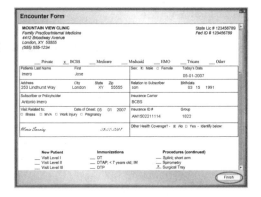

Important: The following instructions and notations will help as you go through the insurance form and make notations of errors.

It is indicated on Jose Imero's registration form that he is a student. For this exercise, consider his status as full-time student.

- Boxes 24 I and J should be left blank.
- For Box 25, you can locate the federal tax ID number on the Encounter Form at the top right-hand side.
- For Box 31, the office will file the claim the same date as the service was provided.
- For Box 33, the NPI number is 1234567899.

1. Below, list any errors you found as you reviewed Jose Imero's insurance claim form.

1500

HEALTH INSURANCE CLAIM FORM

APPROVED BY NATIONAL UNIFORM CLAIM COMMITTEE 08/05

CARRIER

☐☐ PICA   PICA ☐☐

1. MEDICARE ☐ (Medicare #) MEDICAID ☐ (Medicaid #) TRICARE CHAMPUS ☐ (Sponsor's SSN) CHAMPVA ☐ (Member ID#) GROUP HEALTH PLAN ☒ (SSN or ID) FECA BLK LUNG ☐ (SSN) OTHER ☐ (ID)	1a. INSURED'S I.D. NUMBER (For Program in Item 1) YAM 150221114

2. PATIENT'S NAME (Last Name, First Name, Middle Initial)
Imero, Jose

3. PATIENT'S BIRTH DATE MM 03 DD 15 YY 91   SEX M ☒ F ☐

4. INSURED'S NAME (Last Name, First Name, Middle Initial)
IMERO ANTONIO

5. PATIENT'S ADDRESS (No., Street)
253 Lindhurst Way

6. PATIENT RELATIONSHIP TO INSURED
Self ☐ Spouse ☐ Child ☒ Other ☐

7. INSURED'S ADDRESS (No., Street)
4628 Mission Way

CITY **London**   STATE **XY**

8. PATIENT STATUS
Single ☐ Married ☐ Other ☐

CITY **Trumball**   STATE **YZ**

ZIP CODE **55555**   TELEPHONE (Include Area Code) **(555) 555-5455**

Employed ☐ Full-Time Student ☐ Part-Time Student ☒

ZIP CODE **99999**   TELEPHONE (Include Area Code) **(555) 555-7878**

9. OTHER INSURED'S NAME (Last Name, First Name, Middle Initial)

10. IS PATIENT'S CONDITION RELATED TO:

11. INSURED'S POLICY GROUP OR FECA NUMBER
1822

a. OTHER INSURED'S POLICY OR GROUP NUMBER

a. EMPLOYMENT? (Current or Previous)
☐ YES ☒ NO

a. INSURED'S DATE OF BIRTH MM 12 DD 12 YY 74   SEX M ☒ F ☐

b. OTHER INSURED'S DATE OF BIRTH MM DD YY   SEX M ☐ F ☐

b. AUTO ACCIDENT?   PLACE (State)
☐ YES ☒ NO

b. EMPLOYER'S NAME OR SCHOOL NAME
Sunshine Foods

c. EMPLOYER'S NAME OR SCHOOL NAME

c. OTHER ACCIDENT?
☒ YES ☐ NO

c. INSURANCE PLAN NAME OR PROGRAM NAME
Blue Cross/Blue Shield

d. INSURANCE PLAN NAME OR PROGRAM NAME

10d. RESERVED FOR LOCAL USE

d. IS THERE ANOTHER HEALTH BENEFIT PLAN?
☐ YES ☒ NO   *If yes,* return to and complete item 9 a-d.

READ BACK OF FORM BEFORE COMPLETING & SIGNING THIS FORM.

12. PATIENT'S OR AUTHORIZED PERSON'S SIGNATURE I authorize the release of any medical or other information necessary to process this claim. I also request payment of government benefits either to myself or to the party who accepts assignment below.

SIGNED **Signature on File**   DATE

13. INSURED'S OR AUTHORIZED PERSON'S SIGNATURE I authorize payment of medical benefits to the undersigned physician or supplier for services described below.

SIGNED **Signature on File**

PATIENT AND INSURED INFORMATION

14. DATE OF CURRENT MM 05 DD 01 YY 07   ILLNESS (First symptom) OR INJURY (Accident) OR PREGNANCY(LMP)

15. IF PATIENT HAS HAD SAME OR SIMILAR ILLNESS. GIVE FIRST DATE MM DD YY

16. DATES PATIENT UNABLE TO WORK IN CURRENT OCCUPATION
FROM MM DD YY   TO MM DD YY

17. NAME OF REFERRING PROVIDER OR OTHER SOURCE
17a.
17b. NPI

18. HOSPITALIZATION DATES RELATED TO CURRENT SERVICES
FROM MM DD YY   TO MM DD YY

19. RESERVED FOR LOCAL USE

20. OUTSIDE LAB? ☐ YES ☒ NO $ CHARGES

21. DIAGNOSIS OR NATURE OF ILLNESS OR INJURY (Relate Items 1, 2, 3 or 4 to Item 24E by Line)
1. Open Wound L foot 8 cm w/ complications
2.
3.
4.

22. MEDICAID RESUBMISSION CODE   ORIGINAL REF. NO.

23. PRIOR AUTHORIZATION NUMBER

24. A. DATE(S) OF SERVICE From MM DD YY To MM DD YY	B. PLACE OF SERVICE	C. EMG	D. PROCEDURES, SERVICES, OR SUPPLIES (Explain Unusual Circumstances) CPT/HCPCS | MODIFIER	E. DIAGNOSIS POINTER	F. $ CHARGES	G. DAYS OR UNITS	H. EPSDT Family Plan	I. ID. QUAL	J. RENDERING PROVIDER ID. #
1	05 05 07 05 01 07	11		Est. visit, Level II	laceration	45 00	1	N	NPI
2				Tetanus	laceration	15 00	1	N	NPI
3				Immun. Single	laceration	25 00	1	N	NPI
4				Surgical Tray	laceration	15 00	1	N	NPI
5				Wound Repair	laceration	175 00	1	N	NPI
6									NPI

25. FEDERAL TAX I.D. NUMBER   SSN EIN
123456789   ☐ ☒

26. PATIENT'S ACCOUNT NO.

27. ACCEPT ASSIGNMENT? (For govt. claims, see back)
☒ YES ☐ NO

28. TOTAL CHARGE $ **275 00**

29. AMOUNT PAID $ **25 00**

30. BALANCE DUE $ **250 00**

31. SIGNATURE OF PHYSICIAN OR SUPPLIER INCLUDING DEGREES OR CREDENTIALS (I certify that the statements on the reverse apply to this bill and are made a part thereof.)
SOF
SIGNED   DATE **05012007**

32. SERVICE FACILITY LOCATION INFORMATION
44 BROADWAY
LONDON, XY, 55555
a. NPI   b.

33. BILLING PROVIDER INFO & PH # ( )
NATHAN HAYLER MD
4412 BROADWAY
LONDON, XY, 55555
a. **1234567899** b.

PHYSICIAN OR SUPPLIER INFORMATION

NUCC Instruction Manual available at: www.nucc.org   APPROVED OMB-0938-0999 FORM CMS-1500 (08/05)

LESSON 10

Bookkeeping

/⊙⊙ **Reading Assignment:** Chapter 22—Professional Fees, Billing, and Collecting
- How Fees Are Determined
- Bookkeeping Computations Used on Patient Accounts
- Comparison of Manual and Computerized Bookkeeping Systems
- Special Bookkeeping Entries
- Payment Options
- Collection Techniques
- Using Outside Collection Assistance

Chapter 23—Banking Services and Procedures

Chapter 24—Financial and Practice Management
- What Is Accounting?

Patients: All

Learning Objectives:

- Post daily entries on the day sheet and prepare bank deposits at the end of the day.
- Process credit balances, NSF checks, and checks from collection agencies.
- Process credit balances and complete the necessary steps to process a refund, including preparation of a check.
- Reconcile a bank statement.
- Maintain a petty cash fund.
- Discuss the maintenance of records for accounting and banking purposes.
- Discuss the importance of managing accounts payable promptly.

Overview:

In this lesson the basic bookkeeping procedures will be accomplished. All patients will be added to the day sheet, along with the payments and the NSF checks received in today's mail. A deposit record will be prepared. The steps for the reconciliation of the bank statement and maintenance of records for accounting purposes will also be covered.

111

Exercise 1

Online Activity—Posting Charges to Ledger Cards

30 minutes

- Sign in to Mountain View Clinic.
- Select **Jade Wong** from the patient list.

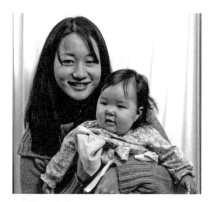

- On the office map, highlight and click on **Billing and Coding**.

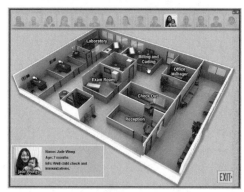

- In the Billing and Coding office, select **Encounter Form** to review the services that will be billed for Jade's visit.

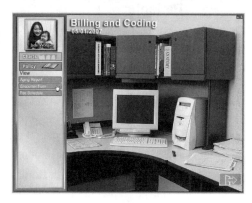

1. a. Using the Encounter Form for Jade Wong, begin completing the blank ledger card below.
   b. In the column marked Professional Service, list each individual service provided, but do not enter any fee or balance information.
   c. After the last service has been entered, be sure to record that the copay was collected and enter the amount in the Payment column.

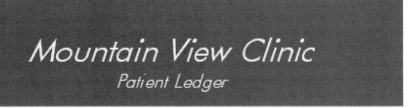

Patient Name:
Insurance Type:

Date	Professional Service	Fee ($)	Payment ($)	Adj. ($)	Prev. Bal. ($)	New Balance ($)
Totals						

• Click **Finish** to return to Billing and Coding.
• Now click on **Fee Schedule** to review the amount Mountain View Clinic charges for various services and procedures.

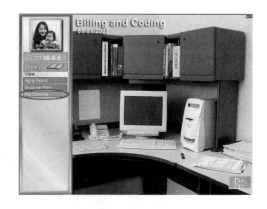

• Again using the ledger card on the previous page, fill in the fees charged for the listed services and calculate the balances.

Important: The balance should be corrected line by line as each service or payment is added or subtracted.

2. After filling in the services, fees, and payments for Jade's current visit, should the ledger card be totaled as indicated at the bottom of the card? Refer to the textbook, if needed, and explain your answer.

3. How did the medical assistant know what Jade's copay was?

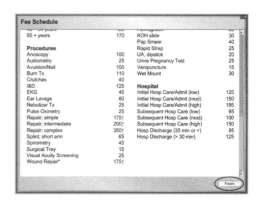 • Click **Finish** to close the Fee Schedule; then click the exit arrow to leave Billing and Coding.

• On the Summary Menu, click on **Return to Map** and continue to the next exercise.

Exercise 2

Online Activity—Posting Entries to a Day Sheet

 60 minutes

1. In this activity you will post charges and payments for the patients who were seen in the office today, using the day sheet on the next page. Note that the distribution columns are used to indicate which physician, Dr. Hayler or Dr. Meyer, provided care to the patient. The amount of money the patient paid should be written in one of those columns in addition to the payment column.

   a. In the Patient Name column on the blank day sheet on the next page, list the patients in the following order: Jade Wong, Louise Parlet, Hu Huang, Rhea Davison, Jesus Santo, Jean Deere, Tristan Tsosie, Wilson Metcalf, Renee Anderson, Jose Imero, Shaunti Begay, Janet Jones, Kevin McKinzie, John R. Simmons, and Teresa Hernandez.

   b. Select Jade Wong from the patient list. Then click on **Check Out** on the office map. Once in the Check Out area, open the **Encounter Form**.

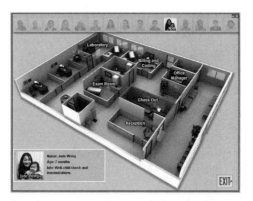

   c. Using one line per patient, complete each column on the day sheet using the Total Charges, Previous Balance, and Amount Received information listed on the Encounter Form. Refer back to the ledger card in Exercise 1 to confirm your totals. (*Note:* Unlike the ledger card, the Professional Service column on the day sheet is a summary description of the visit.)

   d. For the purposes of this exercise, also make a note next to each patient's name to indicate whether the patient paid by cash, check, or credit card. If payment was made by check, include the check number.

   e. Repeat the above steps by selecting each patient listed on the day sheet and opening his or her Encounter Form at Check Out. As you finish each patient's portion of the day sheet, click **Finish** to close the Encounter Form. Click the exit arrow to leave Check Out and **Return to Map** to select the next patient.

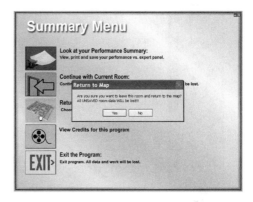

   f. When you finish recording the information for the last patient on the list, remain at the office map to continue with the next question.

Mountain View Clinic
Daysheet

Date	Professional Service	Fee	Payment	Adjustment	New Balance	Old Balance	Patient's Name	Distribution	
								Dr. Hayler	Dr. Meyer
TOTALS									TOTALS

→ • From the office map, click on **Reception**. (The selected patient should be Teresa Hernandez, the last patient on the list in question 1.)

• At the Reception desk, click on **Incoming Mail** to view the day's correspondence.

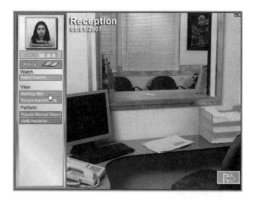

2. a. View each piece of incoming mail; then on the blank day sheet on the next page, record any payments received by the clinic and any charges paid by the clinic in the appropriate columns.

b. Be sure to include a description of the payment/charge and the patient's name.

c. For the purposes of this exercise, make a note of the bank and check number next to the name of any patient who paid by check.

d. To complete the remaining columns, first click **Finish** to close the mail.

e. Next, click the exit arrow and **Return to Map**.

f. Click on **Office Manager** and then on **Day Sheet** (under View) to find any previous balance information for the patients whose accounts were updated from the mail received.

g. Mark Bonsel's previous account balance was zero ("0") before you received the NSF check. The NSF check shows that it was paid on April 7, 2007, but it does not indicate what it was for, other than a balance. Assume it was for a level II new patient visit, which would be $65.00 on the date of April 7, 2007.

Note: A copy of Sarah Anita's EOB from Blue Cross/Blue Shield was received in the mail. The insurance payment and adjustment were already posted on the day sheet and on her ledger in the office manager's section of the Office. The copy of the EOB in the mail will not need to be posted again.

Recalculate the balance and record it in the New Balance column.

Mountain View Clinic
Daysheet

Date	Professional Service	Fee	Payment	Adjustment	New Balance	Old Balance	Patient's Name	Distribution Dr. Hayler	Distribution Dr. Meyer
TOTALS								TOTALS	

• Click **Finish** and continue to the next exercise.

Exercise 3

  Writing Activity—Preparing a Bank Deposit

  15 minutes

Using the information recorded in the completed day sheets in Exercise 2, you will now prepare a bank deposit (both front and back) for the accounts receivable for the day. Be sure the total on the deposit slip balances with the total of receivables on the day sheet.

1. Below, complete the front side of the deposit slip.

DEPOSIT SLIP

Clarion National Bank
90 Grape Vine Road
London, XY 55555-0001

Mountain View Clinic
4412 Broadway
London, XY 55555

Date: _____

CASH			TOTAL
	Currency	$_____	
	Coin	$_____	$_____
	Total Cash		$_____
CHECKS	See other side for detail		$_____
- CASH REC'D			$_____
NET DEPOSIT			$_____

_____
SIGN HERE IN TELLER'S PRESENCE FOR CASH RECEIVED

2. Below, complete the back portion of the bank deposit slip. (*Note:* The bank number cannot be obtained from the day sheet. For the purposes of this exercise, use the check number as a substitute.)

BANK DEPOSIT DETAIL

PAYMENTS

BANK NUMBER	BY CHECK OR PMO		BY COIN OR CURRENCY		CREDIT CARD	
TOTALS						
CURRENCY						
COIN						
CHECKS						
CREDIT CARDS						
TOTAL RECEIPTS						
LESS CREDIT CARD $						
TOTAL DEPOSIT						
DEPOSIT DATE _____						

Exercise 4

Online Activity—Processing a Credit Balance

20 minutes

- Remain in the manager's office and click on **Day Sheet**. (*Note:* If you have exited the manager's office and are at the office map, click on **Office Manager** and then click on **Day Sheet**.)

1. Two patients listed on the day sheet have overpaid, which resulted in a credit balance denoted by a parenthesis around the amount that was overpaid. Betsy Dunworthy overpaid by $20.00, and her refund was already processed. What is the name of the other patient who should receive a refund, and how much money should he receive?

2. Using the blank check below, process the outstanding refund for payment.

173975		MOUNTAIN VIEW CLINIC	173975

4412 Broadway
London, XY 55555

94-72/1224

Date: _____

DATE: _____

TO: _____

FOR: _____

Pay to the order of: _____

ACCOUNT NO. _____

_____ Dollars $ [   ]

AMOUNT PAID $ _____

Clarion National Bank
  Member FDIC
90 Grape Vine Road
London, XY 55555-0001

_____
Authorized Signature

⑈ 005503 ⑈ 46782011 ⑈ 678800470

→ - Click **Finish** to return to the manager's office.

Exercise 5

Online Activity—Maintaining Petty Cash Fund

30 minutes

- In the office manager's office, click on **Petty Cash Log**. (*Note:* If you have exited the office manager's office and are at the office map, click on **Office Manager** and select **Petty Cash Log**.)

1. Petty cash was used to pay for the mailing of a certified letter. What are the receipt number and date from this transaction?

2. On 5-1-07, the administrative medical assistant was asked to obtain soft drinks for an office celebration to be held that afternoon. These were bought at Sav-A-Grocery for the amount of $24.56. She also mailed a large package at the post office. The cost for mailing the package was $15.08. Using the form below, fill out the first petty cash voucher.

Date: _____   No.: __109__

PETTY CASH VOUCHER

For: _____

Charge to: _____

_____

Approved by: Received by:

_____   _____

Authorized Signature

---

3. Now fill out the second petty cash voucher.

Date: _____   No.: __110__

PETTY CASH VOUCHER

For: _____

Charge to: _____

_____

Approved by: Received by:

_____   _____
Authorized Signature

4. Using the completed petty cash vouchers from questions 2 and 3, update the petty cash log below accordingly. Be sure to distribute the expenses to the proper expense column.

NO.	DATE	DESCRIPTION	AMOUNT	OFFICE EXP.	AUTO.	MISC.	BALANCE
	2/16/2007	Fund Established (check #217)					200.00
101	2/24/2007	Certified Letter	3.74	3.74			196.26
102	3/1/2007	Staff Meeting/Lunch	24.60			24.60	171.66
103	3/6/2007	Coffee	4.32			4.32	167.34
104	3/8/2007	Tympanic Thermometer	38.00	38.00			129.34
105	3/8/2007	Parking Fee	6.00		6.00		123.34
106	4/1/2007	Staff Meeting/Lunch	27.43			27.43	95.91
107	4/13/2007	Miscellaneous Supplies	9.01	9.01			86.90
108	4/21/2007	Patient Birthday Cards	12.17	12.17			74.73

5. Office policy states that petty cash should be replenished when the amount falls below $50. Use the blank check below to replenish the petty cash fund to the full $200 balance as required by office policy. Then, using the updated petty cash log in question 4, verify the petty cash fund balances by totaling all the columns, and add this transaction to the log.

173976

DATE:	
TO:	
FOR:	
ACCOUNT NO.	
AMOUNT PAID	$

MOUNTAIN VIEW CLINIC 173976
4412 Broadway
London, XY 55555   94-72/1224

Date: _____

Pay to the order of: _____

_____ Dollars $ _____

Clarion National Bank
            Member FDIC
90 Grape Vine Road
London, XY 55555-0001   _____
                                         Authorized Signature

||⁢ 005503 ||⁢ 46782011 ||⁢ 678800470

➡ • Click **Finish** to return to the manager's office.

• Click the exit arrow; from the Summary Menu, select **Return to Map**.

• On the office map, select **Jose Imero** from the patient list and click on **Check Out**.

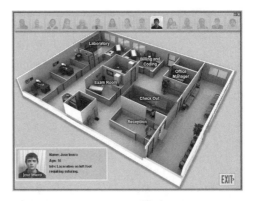

• At the Check Out desk, select **Patient Check Out** (under Watch) to view the video.

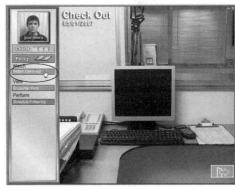

6. What are the ethical implications of Kristin asking another medical assistant for money from petty cash?

- Click **Close** to return to the Check Out desk.
- Click the exit arrow; from the Summary Menu, select **Return to Map**.

Exercise 6

Online Activity—Managing Accounts Payable

30 minutes

- Using any patient from the patient list, click on **Reception** on the office map.
- Select **Incoming Mail** (under View) and review pieces 8 and 9.

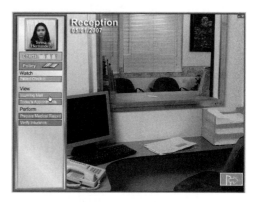

1. Indicate whether each of the following statements is true or false.

   a. _____ When accounts payable arrive, the date for payment with discounts should be noted.

   b. _____ It really does not matter what day of the month an accounts payable payment is made, as long as it is paid before the next billing cycle.

   c. _____ Invoices should be marked with the date and check number, as well as the initials of the person preparing the check.

   d. _____ All accounts payables should be checked against invoices and packing slips before payment is made to ensure that everything ordered was received.

   e. _____ All vendors will present invoices before payment is due.

2. Which of the following information does the accounts payable person need to correctly process and post the payment of the invoices (pieces 8 and 9 of the incoming mail)? Select all that apply.

_____ Invoice number

_____ Company name

_____ Name of the customer service representative

_____ Date of the check

_____ Account number

_____ Company address

_____ Company phone number

_____ Name of the company's bank

_____ Company's bank account number

_____ Type of expense

_____ Amount of the check

_____ Invoice date

_____ Check number

- Click **Finish** to close the mail and return to the Reception desk.
- Click the exit arrow; from the Summary Menu, select **Return to Map**.

Exercise 7

Online Activity—Reconciling a Bank Statement

🕐 30 minutes

The clinic's bank statement arrives in today's mail. This is found in the manager's office. She is extremely busy and asks that you take the time to reconcile the statement for her.

- On the office map, click on **Office Manager** to enter the manager's office. (*Note:* For this task, it does not matter which patient is selected. You may continue with Jose Imero from the previous exercise.)
- From the menu on the left, select **Bank Statement**.

1. a. Using the check ledger below, review the bank statement and check off each deposit, check, withdrawal, ATM transaction, or credit listed on the statement.

   b. If the statement shows any interest paid to the account, service charges, bank fees, automatic payments, or ATM transactions withdrawn from the account that are not listed on the check ledger, make an entry for those items now and recalculate the account balance in the ledger.

No.	Date	Description	Payment/ Debit	Ref	Deposit/ Credit	Balance
1216	4/5/2007	Rocke Medical	$625.00			$9,264.35
1217	4/5/2007	Wal Store	$38.46			$9,225.89
1218	4/6/2007	Lorenz Equipment	$1006.00			$8,219.89
1219	4/8/2007	Office Station	$199.43			$8,020.46
	4/10/2007	Dep. Daily Trans			$1,050.00	$10,833.46
1220	4/10/2007	West Electric	$93.99			$7,926.47
	4/12/2007	Dep. Daily Trans			$2,008.00	$9,934.47
1221	4/12/2007	Office Depot	$102.01			$9,832.46
1222	4/12/2007	Video Inc.	$49.00			$9,783.46
	4/15/2007	Dep. Daily Trans			$1,002.00	$11,835.46
1223	4/17/2007	Bonus	$200.00			$12,560.46
1224	4/17/2007	Bonus	$200.00			$12,360.46
1225	4/17/2007	Bonus	$200.00			$12,160.46
	4/20/2007	Dep. Daily Trans			$925.00	$12,760.46
1226	4/21/2007	Jamison Medical	$2,024.00			$10,136.26
1227	4/22/2007	Healthy Living Magazine	$32.95			$10,103.31
1228	4/22/2007	Greater London Electric	$422.00			$9,681.31
1229	4/24/2007	Office Station	$344.70			$9,336.61
1230	4/25/2007	Summer Oxygen	$230.99			$9,105.62
	4/27/2007	Dep. Daily Trans			$1,550.00	$10,655.62

2. Now complete the bank reconciliation worksheet below.

THIS WORKSHEET IS PROVIDED TO HELP YOU BALANCE YOUR ACCOUNT

1. Go through your register and mark each check, withdrawal, Express ATM transaction, payment, deposit or other credit listed on your statement. Be sure that your register shows any interest paid into your account, and any service charges, bank fees, automatic payments, or Express Transfers withdrawn from your account during this statement period.

2. Using the chart below, list any outstanding checks, Express ATM withdrawals, payments or any other withdrawals (including any from previous months) that are listed in your register but are not shown on this statement.

3. Balance your account by filling in the spaces below.

ITEMS OUTSTANDING	
NUMBER	**AMOUNT**
TOTAL	

ENTER

The ENDING BALANCE shown on this statement ------------------------------- $ _____ __

ADD

Any deposits listed in your register or $ _____ __
transfers into your account which are $ _____ __
not shown on this statement $ _____ __
          +$ _____ __

TOTAL----------------------------------+ $ _____ __

CALCULATE THE SUBTOTAL --- $ _____ __

SUBTRACT

The total outstanding checks and
Withdrawals from the chart at the left ------------------------------------- $ _____ __

CALCULATE THE ENDING BALANCE

This amount should be the same as
The current balance shown in your
Check register --- $ _____ __

Payroll Procedures

👓 **Reading Assignment:** Chapter 24—Financial and Practice Management
  • Payroll Records

Patients: None

Learning Objectives:

- Process the employee payroll.
- Locate federal tax withholding resources by using the Internet

Overview:

For administrative medical assistants, the task of preparing an employee payroll may be a routine function. This lesson will give you practice in preparing a payroll for employees.

Exercise 1

Online Activity—Processing Payroll

  20 minutes

- Sign in to Mountain View Clinic.
- On the office map, highlight and click on **Office Manager** to enter the manager's office.
  (*Note:* You do not need to select a patient for this exercise.)

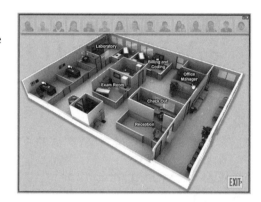

- Click on **Payroll Forms** to view the office payroll records.

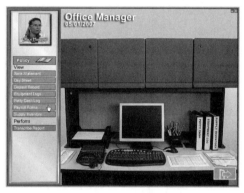

- The time sheet for employee Cathy Wright will appear first. Review and confirm that the number of hours has been calculated correctly.
- Next, click on the down arrow next to Person and select **Susan Bronski**.
- Review Susan Bronski's time sheet and confirm the calculations for the number of hours she worked.

1. Cathy Wright's total number of hours worked: _____

   Susan Bronski's total number of hours worked: _____

2. Cathy Wright has been employed by the clinic for 10 years. Her salary is $18.00 per hour for the first 80 hours and $27.00 per hour for any hours over 80 during the 2-week pay period. Compute the gross pay for Cathy for the 2-week period.

3. Susan Bronski is a relatively new employee who is making $15.00 per hour for the first 80 hours and $20 per hour for hours over 80. Compute the gross pay for Susan for the 2-week period.

- Now review the W-4 form filled out by each employee.
- To view Cathy Wright's W-4 form, first make sure her name is selected from the drop-down menu next to Person. Next, click on the down arrow next to Form and select **W-4**. Review her form.
- To view Susan Bronski's W-4 form, select her name from the drop-down menu next to Person.

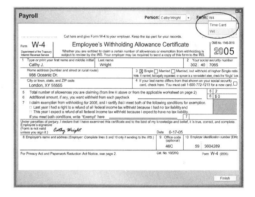

4. Cathy Wright elected to have her federal taxes withheld under which designation?

_____ Single

_____ Married

_____ Married, but withhold at the higher single rate

5. The number of allowances claimed by Cathy Wright is _____.

6. Did Cathy Wright elect to have any additional money withheld from her paycheck for federal taxes? If yes, how much?

7. Susan Bronski will have her federal taxes withheld under which designation?

_____ Single

_____ Married

_____ Married, but withhold at the higher single rate

8. The number of allowances claimed by Susan Bronski is _____.

9. Did Susan Bronski elect to have any additional money withheld from her paycheck for federal taxes? If yes, how much?

Exercise 2

Writing Activity—Calculating Net Pay

30 minutes

The IRS updates the federal tax tables each year. The tables we are using for this activity are 2010 tables for Single and Married Persons Biweekly Payroll (you will choose which table to use based on the employees filing status). Go to the Evolve course website. Click on Course Documents to view the 2010 tax tables. If you are instructed by your teacher to obtain the most recent copy of the schedules, go to the IRS website at www.irs.gov. Each state may have its own amount for the state withholding, but for this exercise we will use 1%.

1. Calculate the federal withholding allowance for Cathy Wright and Susan Bronski.

Total withholding allowance (federal) for Cathy Wright: _____

Total withholding allowance (federal) for Susan Bronski: _____

2. Now subtract the total withholding allowance from each employee's gross pay to calculate the adjusted gross pay.

   Cathy Wright's adjusted gross pay: _____

   Susan Bronski's adjusted gross pay: _____

3. Account for the following additional deductions for Cathy Wright: Medicare = 1.45%, Social Security = 6.2%, Health Insurance = $125 per pay, State Income Tax = 1%, Retirement Plan = $150 per pay.

Federal Income Tax	
Medicare	
Social Security	
Health Insurance	
State Income Tax	
Retirement Savings Plan	

4. What is the net pay for Cathy Wright? _____

5. a. Using the correct tax table, calculate the correct deductions for Susan Bronski, who will file as head of household.

b. Account for the following additional deductions for Susan Bronski: Medicare = 1.45%, Social Security = 6.2%, Health Insurance = $175 per pay, State Income Tax = 1%, Savings Plan = $50 per pay period, Additional Tax Withholding from W-4 = $190.00.

Federal Income Tax	
Medicare	
Social Security	
Health Insurance	
State Income Tax	
Retirement Savings Plan	
Additional Tax Withholding	

6. What is the net pay for Susan Bronski? _____

Exercise 3

 Online Activity—Writing the Check for Payroll

 15 minutes

You are now ready to prepare and issue the payroll checks for Cathy Wright and Susan Bronski. To obtain the correct ending date for the pay period, return to the employees' time sheets by clicking on **Payroll Forms** in the manager's office. Date the checks for the Monday following the end of the pay period.

1. Prepare Cathy Wright's payroll check below.

PERIOD ENDING	EARNINGS			DEDUCTIONS										NET PAY
HOURS WORKED REG. OT	REGULAR	OVERTIME	TOTAL	FEDERAL INCOME TAX	FICA TAX	STATE INCOME TAX	SDI TAX	HEALTH INS.	SAVINGS	MEDICARE	MISC. DED.		TOTAL DED.	AMOUNT

CHECK # 173977   Employee:

- -

MOUNTAIN VIEW CLINIC   173977
4412 Broadway
London, XY 55555   94-72/1224

                                                          Date: _____

Pay to the order of: _____

_____ Dollars | $ |

Clarion National Bank
    Member FDIC
90 Grape Vine Road
London, XY 55555-0001   _____
                                                   Authorized Signature

||⌐ 005503 ||⌐ ⌐4678201l ||⌐ 678800470

2. Prepare Susan Bronski's payroll check below.

PERIOD ENDING	EARNINGS			DEDUCTIONS								NET PAY	
HOURS WORKED REG. OT	REGULAR	OVERTIME	TOTAL	FEDERAL INCOME TAX	FICA TAX	STATE INCOME TAX	SDI TAX	HEALTH INS.	SAVINGS	MEDICARE	MISC. DED.	TOTAL DED.	AMOUNT

CHECK # 173978   **Employee:**

MOUNTAIN VIEW CLINIC   173978
4412 Broadway
London, XY 55555   94-72/1224

                                                          Date: _____

Pay to the order of: _____

_____ Dollars | $ |

Clarion National Bank
  Member FDIC
90 Grape Vine Road
London, XY 55555-0001   _____
                                                Authorized Signature

   ||⁛ 005503 ||⁛ 446782011 ||⁛ 678800470

LESSON 12

Standard Precautions and Biohazardous Materials

Reading Assignment: Chapter 27—Infection Control
- OSHA Standards for the Healthcare Setting

Patients: Shaunti Begay, Hu Huang, Tristan Tsosie

Learning Objectives:

- Recognize what materials are biohazardous.
- Indicate the proper disposal of used medical equipment and supplies.
- Identify the proper practice of standard precautions.
- Understand how to apply OSHA standards.
- Apply critical thinking skills to answer questions regarding biohazardous waste.
- Understand the importance of an infection control plan and its impact on preventing the spread of disease in the medical facility.

Overview:

In this lesson standard precautions (as dictated by OSHA regulations) will be discussed. You will learn to distinguish acceptable practices from those procedures that could cause injury to patients and staff. Included in the practice of universal precautions are standard precautions, which include the appropriate disposal of biohazardous waste. (*Note:* Although medical asepsis, including handwashing, is an important factor in infection control, this topic is covered in another lesson and will not be addressed here.)

Exercise 1

Online Activity—Infection Control in the Medical Office Using OSHA Standards

20 minutes

- Sign in to Mountain View Clinic.
- From the patient list, select **Shaunti Begay**.

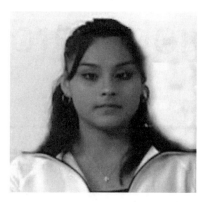

- On the office map, click to enter the **Exam Room**. Inside the Exam Room, click on **Policy** to open the Policy Manual.

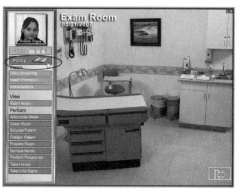

- In the Policy Manual search box, type "OSHA" and click twice on the magnifying glass to review the relevant section.

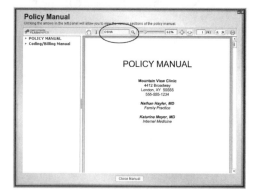

- Read the section of the Policy Manual on OSHA Bloodborne Pathogens.

1. Name four body fluids that would be considered biohazardous waste in this medical office.

    (1)

    (2)

    (3)

    (4)

Critical Thinking Question

2. What additional body secretion is not included in the list of biohazardous waste?

3. To what does the term *universal precaution* refer?

4. What are work practice controls?

5. What are engineering controls?

6. What does PPE stand for?

7. Does OSHA have any directions for maintaining an examination room? If so, what is included in the directions?

→ • Click on **Close** to exit the Policy Manual.
  • Remain in the Exam Room and continue to Exercise 2.

Exercise 2

 Online Activity—Application of OSHA Standards

 30 minutes

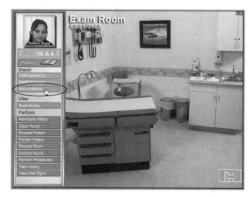

• In this exercise we will continue with Shaunti Begay's visit to the clinic. (*Note:* If you have exited the program, sign in again to Mountain View Clinic, select Shaunti Begay, and go to the Exam Room.)

• From the Exam Room menu, select **Immunization** and watch the video.

• Stop or pause the video at the first fadeout before answering the following questions.

1. Did the medical assistant wear the proper PPE for giving an injection? Explain your answer.

2. Did the medical assistant properly handle the disposal of the gloves and waste from the injection?

3. Where did the medical assistant dispose of the used needle and syringe?

4. What engineering controls did you see in the video?

- Click **Close** to end the video and return to the Exam Room.
- Click on the exit arrow to leave the Exam Room.
- From the Summary Menu, select **Return to Map**.

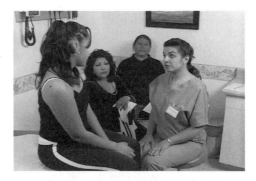

- Select **Hu Huang** from the patient list.

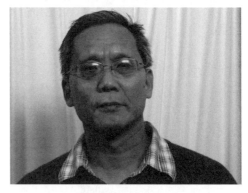

- Click on **Reception** on the office map.

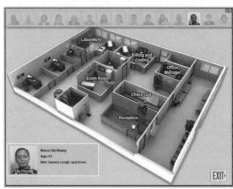

- From the Reception area, click on **Patient Check-In** to watch a video of Hu Huang.

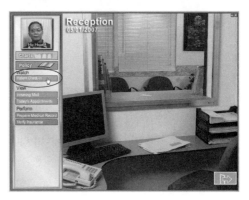

5. Mr. Huang has a productive cough when he approaches the Reception area. He lays a contaminated tissue on the counter just before Kristin takes him to a room. Should she have left the area without disinfecting the counter? Explain your answer.

6. Explain the proper disposal of contaminated tissues.

7. Which of the following are proper steps in infection control that should be observed during the check-in of Mr. Huang? Select all that apply.

_____ Provide tissues as shown in the video.

_____ Allow Mr. Huang to stay in the waiting room.

_____ Throw the tissue in the trash at the desk so that the contamination cannot spread.

_____ Apply gloves before handling the used tissues.

_____ Provide Mr. Huang with a means of disposing of the used tissues in biohazard waste.

_____ Wash hands after disinfecting the counter.

_____ Don a gown and mask when caring for Mr. Huang.

8. Based on the video you watched, how do you think the patients in the waiting room probably felt when the medical assistant stated that Hu Huang might have an infectious disease that could be given to the other patients? Do you think Kristin handled the check-in in an ethical manner? Explain your answer.

9. Suppose Kristin had not put the patient in the examination room. Would you expect patients to verbally complain about Mr. Huang's persistent cough? Would there be times when you could not put a patient into a separate room?

10. Indicate whether each of the following statements is true or false.

    a. _____ Because Mr. Huang laid his contaminated tissue on the counter, OSHA standards would require that Kristin disinfect the counter before allowing another patient to register.

    b. _____ Ideally, after Mr. Huang laid his tissue on the counter, Kristin should have donned gloves and removed the tissue before moving the patient to a room.

    c. _____ Ideally, in offices in which patients may have infectious diseases, a biohazard waste bag should be placed at the check-in window for situations similar to what you saw in the video.

    d. _____ Ideally, the check-in desk should have unsterile gloves available for removing biohazardous waste.

    e. _____ Because Kristin did not touch the contaminated tissues, she does not need to sanitize her hands.

    f. _____ The better method of sanitization of Kristin's hands would be washing.

- Click **Close** to exit the video and return to the Reception area.
- Click on the exit arrow and then on **Return to Map**.
- Click on **Exam Room** to enter the patient examination area.
- From the Exam Room menu, select **Exam Notes** (under View) and read the documentation for Hu Huang's visit. Click **Finish** when you are finished.

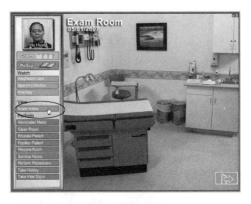

- Now select **Clean Room** (under Perform) and choose the steps that should be taken at the end of Mr. Huang's visit to clean the room before the next patient is seen.
- After making your selections, click **Finish** to return to the Exam Room.

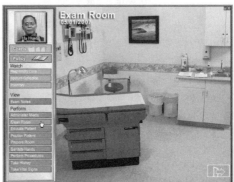

- Click on the exit arrow and select **Look at Your Performance Summary** to check your answers with those of the experts.
- After reviewing your answers, click **Close** and then **Return to Map** to move on to the next exercise.

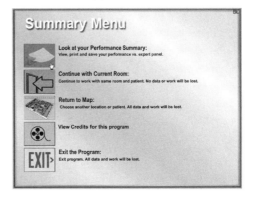

Exercise 3

Online Activity—Applying Knowledge of Federal Regulations (OSHA)

15 minutes

- Select **Tristan Tsosie** from the patient list.
  (*Note:* If you have exited the program, sign in
  again to Mountain View Clinic and select Tristan
  Tsosie from the patient list.)

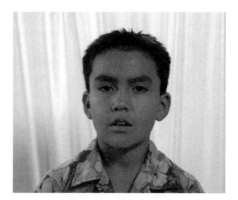

- Click on **Exam Room** on the office map.

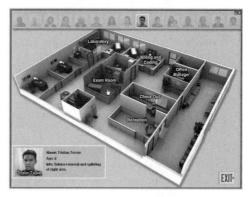

- In the Exam Room, click on **Throat Specimen**
  and watch the video. Observe the infection
  control measures.

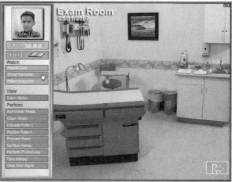

1. Which of the following PPE were used by Cathy when she obtained a throat culture?
   Select all that apply.

   _____ Sterile gloves

   _____ Unsterile gloves

   _____ Face shield

   _____ Sterile gown

   _____ Disposable gown

   _____ Goggles

2. Indicate whether each of the following statements is true or false.

   a. _____ Cathy followed OSHA policy regarding the PPE needed for obtaining a throat culture.

   b. _____ The supplies used to collect the throat specimen should be disposed of in the biohazard waste container.

   c. _____ The gown and mask may be used again with another patient since Tristan did not cough.

   d. _____ The PPE used by Cathy must be provided by her employer.

   e. _____ The biohazard bag is not full at the end of the day, so it is acceptable to add tomorrow's waste and then discard it when the bag is full.

   f. _____ Each medical office must have its own infection control system.

   g. _____ Compliance with OSHA standards is required by law.

3. Do you feel that Cathy handled the use of PPE in an acceptable manner when talking with Tristan? Explain your reasoning.

Handwashing

Reading Assignment: Chapter 27—Infection Control
- Aseptic Techniques: Prevention of Disease Transmission
- Hand Washing
- Role of Medical Assistant in Asepsis

Patients: Jean Deere, Louise Parlet, Kevin McKinzie

Learning Objectives:

- Discuss the rationale for handwashing versus hand sanitization.
- Identify the specific circumstances in which handwashing is appropriate.
- Identify the specific circumstances in which hand sanitization is appropriate.
- Examine the policy manual regarding policies of infection control for this office.
- Use the Internet to research information regarding hand hygiene.

Overview:

Handwashing has been a foundation of infection control for over a century. This practice is still essential today. Handwashing not only protects the patient from cross contamination but also protects the healthcare worker. The CDC has made some changes in its recommendations for handwashing by suggesting the use of alcohol-based hand rubs for certain circumstances. In this lesson we will review the circumstances in which each of these means of hand hygiene should be used.

Exercise 1

Online Activity—Handwashing/Hand Sanitization

40 minutes

- Sign in to Mountain View Clinic.
- From the patient list, click on **Jean Deere**.

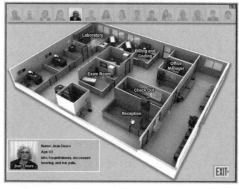

- On the office map, highlight **Reception** and click to enter the Reception area.

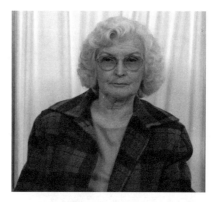

- In the Reception area, click on **Policy** to open the Policy Manual.

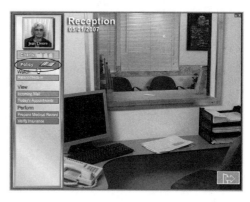

- In the Policy Manual search box, type "handwashing" and click on the magnifying glass to search.

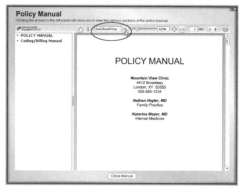

- Read the section of the Policy Manual on handwashing.

- Go to http://www.cdc.gov and search for "hand hygiene" to see recommendations.

- Click on **Close Manual** to return to Reception. To leave the Reception area, click on the exit arrow in the lower right corner of the screen.

- From the Summary Menu, select **Return to Map**.

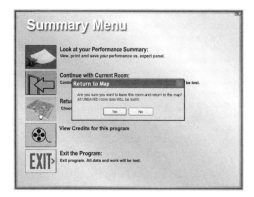

- From the patient list, select **Jesus Santo**, who was the patient seen just before Jean Deere.

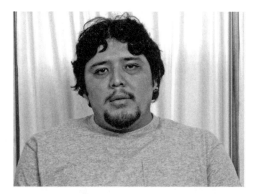

- On the office map, click to enter the **Billing and Coding** area.

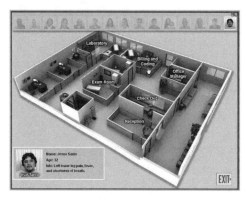

- In the Billing and Coding area, click on **Encounter Form** to review the information for today's visit. Find the diagnosis for Mr. Santo's visit.

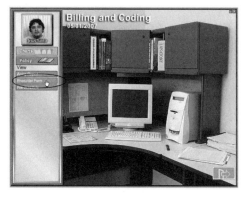

1. Based on the diagnosis listed on the Encounter Form for Mr. Santo and your review of the CDC guidelines for hand hygiene, what would be the correct method of hand hygiene to use between patients?

➤ • Click on **Finish** to close the Encounter Form; then click on the exit arrow to leave the Billing and Coding area.
  • Click on **Return to Map** and select Jean Deere again from the patient list.
  • Click to enter the **Exam Room**.

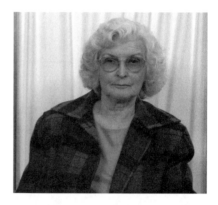

  • From the options under Watch, select **Room Preparation** and observe the video.
  • Click **Close** to return to the Exam Room.

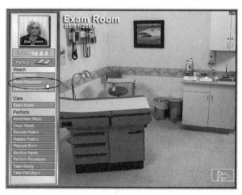

2. Why did the medical assisting extern need to wash her hands before preparing the room for a patient?

3. If the patient seen before Jean Deere did not have a diagnosis with the possibility of disease transmission, what would have been the appropriate form of hand sanitization?

4. If a medical assistant wears gloves, is it necessary to perform hand hygiene when the gloves are removed, prior to working with the next patient?

Thought Question

5. What potential risk do artificial fingernails or natural nails longer than ¼ inch present in the healthcare setting? To assist in your answer, you may go to the CDC website link at http://www.cdc.gov/mmwr/preview/mmwrhtml/rr5116a1.htm to view the CDC's recommendations. Scroll down the page to find Recommendations; then go to number 6.

6. Based on these risks, what are your thoughts about policies regarding prohibiting employees from wearing artificial nails? Develop a short paragraph that would address this in a policy manual.

- From the options under Perform, select **Sanitize Hands** and answer the related question.
- Click on **Finish** and then on the exit arrow to leave the Exam Room.

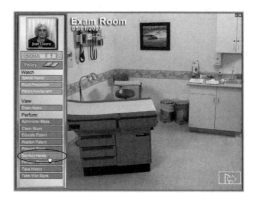

- From the Summary Menu, select **Look at Your Performance Summary**.
- Scroll down the Performance Summary to the Sanitize Hands section and check your answer against that of the experts.
- When you have finished checking your work, click on **Close** and then on **Return to Map**.

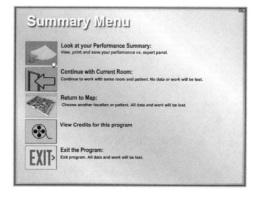

7. Would it have been acceptable for the medical assisting extern to clean the table without gloves if she had sanitized her hands prior to and immediately after disposing of the table paper and gown? Why or why not?

8. After the extern has cleaned the examination table and removed her gloves, what is the appropriate means of hand hygiene?

Exercise 2

Online Activity—Hand Sanitization with Possible Infectious Diseases

15 minutes

- Select **Kevin McKinzie** from the patient list. (*Note:* If you have exited the program, sign in again to Mountain View Clinic and select Kevin McKinzie from the patient list.)

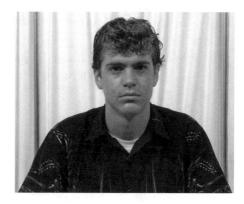

- On the office map, click on **Check Out**.

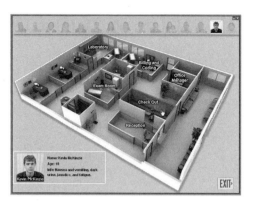

- In the Check Out area, click on **Charts** and then on the **Patient Medical Information** tab. From the drop-down menu, select **1-Progress Notes** to review today's visit.

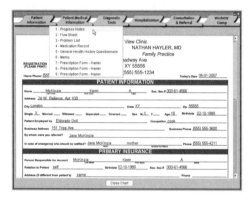

1. What is the possible diagnosis for this patient?

2. With this diagnosis, what would be the safest means of hand hygiene following patient care?

3. _____ According to the CDC, the use of gloves is not necessary when good hand hygiene is used. (True or False)

4. The CDC has recommended the use of alcohol-based hand rubs instead of handwashing in some instances. List two advantages of hand rubs.

5. List three times when handwashing is necessary in the medical office.

    (1)

    (2)

    (3)

6. For what length of time should a handwash be performed at the beginning of the day?

14

Obtaining and Documenting a Health History

Reading Assignment: Chapter 28—Patient Assessment

Patients: Kevin McKinzie, Hu Huang, Tristan Tsosie, Wilson Metcalf

Learning Objectives:

- List the components of the health history and understand the importance of each.
- Identify the questions that should be included during a health history.
- Indicate the accurate method of documenting a health history in a medical record.
- Demonstrate accurate written communication skills.
- Explain the difference between signs and symptoms.
- Differentiate between objective and subjective symptoms.
- Explain the need for confidentiality when obtaining a health history.

Overview:

In this lesson you will learn the proper questions to ask to obtain an accurate health history and the proper method of documenting the information you obtain. Kevin McKinzie is a new patient, whereas Hu Huang is an established patient who has just returned from a visit to China. Both of these patients have specific indications for obtaining an accurate medical history. In both cases, it is especially important for the medical assistant to recognize and respond to verbal and nonverbal communication appropriately.

Exercise 1

  Writing Activity—Background for Obtaining a Health History

30 minutes

1. What components should be included when you obtain a health history?

2. When obtaining a patient's past medical history, why is it important that the medical assistant review this information with the patient rather than just rely on what the patient writes on the form?

3. Why would the physician need to know any previous surgical procedures a patient has undergone and where these procedures were done?

4. What is included in a social history?

5. Why is it important to include educational background in a medical history?

6. Why are environmental factors important to include in a medical history?

7. Define *chief complaint* or *present illness*.

8. While listening to the chief complaint, what should the medical assistant remember to do during the documentation?

9. Subjective symptoms are sometimes simply called _____, whereas

   objective symptoms are called _____. Symptoms of the greatest

   significance are called _____ symptoms.

10. How are subjective symptoms obtained?

11. How are objective symptoms obtained?

12. Why is it important that the medical assistant ask questions of the patient in a private area rather than in the reception area?

Exercise 2

Online Activity—Obtaining a Medical History from a New Patient

30 minutes

- Sign in to Mountain View Clinic.
- From the patient list, select **Kevin McKinzie**.

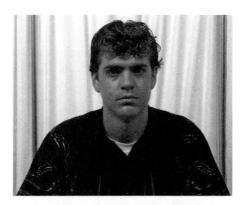

- On the office map, highlight and click on **Reception**.

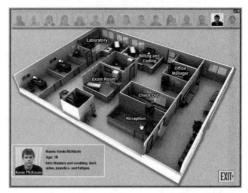

- Under the Watch heading, select **Patient Check-In** to view the video.

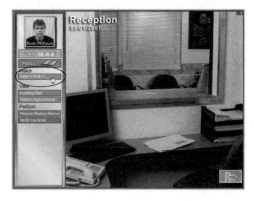

• Click **Close** at the end of the video to return to Reception.

1. Kevin McKinzie brings a history form to the medical office with him. What are the disadvantages of having the patient complete the medical history at home?

2. The administrative medical assistant takes the medical history and places it in a chart without reviewing it for completeness. Is this good practice? Explain your answer.

3. If the history was not complete, would it be appropriate for the medical assistant to gather additional information at the window?

4. Would you have handled the check-in of Mr. McKinzie differently? If yes, explain how. Did the medical assistant respond adequately to the patient's verbal and nonverbal communication?

 • Click the exit arrow at the bottom right of the screen to leave the Reception area.
  • On the Summary Menu, click **Return to Map**.

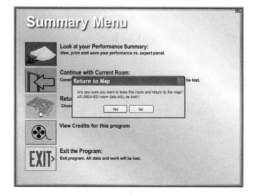

- On the office map, highlight and click on **Exam Room** to continue with Mr. McKinzie's visit.

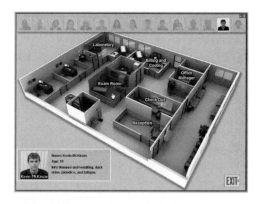

- From the menu on the left, click on **Charts** and select **1-General Health History Questionnaire** from the drop-down menu under the **Patient Medical Information** tab.

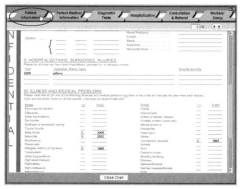

- Using the arrow at the top right of the questionnaire, turn to page 2.
- Thoroughly review the information Mr. McKinzie provided on page 2 of the questionnaire.

5. What is the patient's chief complaint as documented under Current Medical History?

6. What are two areas of Mr. McKinzie's social history that could have a bearing on this illness?

- Again using the arrow at the top of the screen, turn to page 3 of the questionnaire.
- Thoroughly review the information Mr. McKinzie provided regarding his past history.

Critical Thinking Question

7. What, if any, familial history is relevant to his chief complaint?

• Still in the chart, click on the **Patient Information** tab and select **1-Patient Information Form**.

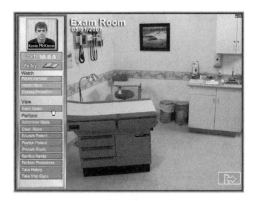

• Read the Patient Information Form to find Mr. McKinzie's type of employment.

• Click **Close Chart** to return to the Exam Room.

• Click on **Exam Notes** (under View) and read the clinical diagnoses as documented by Dr. Hayler.

• Click **Finish** to close the Exam Notes and return to the Exam Room.

8. What are the indications for patient education and infection control for these clinical diagnoses?

 • Click the exit arrow to leave the Exam Room.

• On the Summary Menu, click **Return to Map** and continue to the next exercise.

Exercise 3

 Online Activity—Documentation of the Chief Complaint for an Established Patient

 40 minutes

• From the patient list, select **Hu Huang**. (*Note:* If you have exited the program, sign in again to Mountain View Clinic and select Hu Huang from the patient list.)

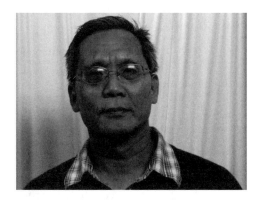

- On the office map, highlight and click on **Exam Room**.

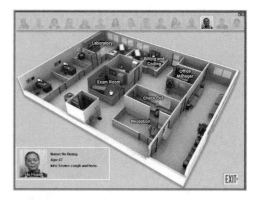

- Under the Watch heading, select **Respiratory Care** to view the video.

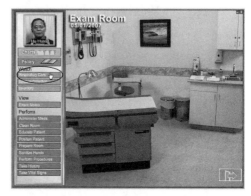

- Click **Close** at the end of the video to return to the Exam Room.
- Click on **Exam Notes** (under View) to read the documentation of Mr. Huang's visit.

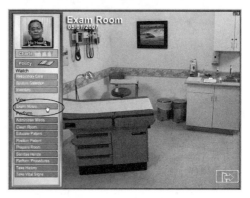

1. What is your assessment of the verbal and nonverbal communication that Charlie conducted with Mr. Huang in the video?

2. Why do you think Charlie seemed a little "stiff" with his body language?

3. What is the chief complaint for Mr. Huang?

4. Which of the symptoms listed are subjective symptoms?

5. What are the objective symptoms?

6. What other information could be placed in the History section of the Progress Notes?

7. Why was it important to obtain the information that Mr. Huang had been in China for several months?

 • Click **Finish** to close the Exam Notes and return to the Exam Room.
   • Open Mr. Huang's **Chart** and select **1-Progress Notes** from the drop-down menu under the **Patient Medical Information** tab.
   • Read the documentation from all of Mr. Huang's previous visits.

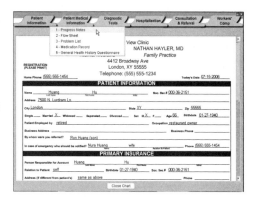

8. After reading the Progress Notes for all his visits, what questions would have been appropriate for the medical assistant to ask Mr. Huang regarding medication compliance?

9. Indicate whether each of the following statements is true or false regarding documentation of patient history in Progress Notes on established patients.

a. _____ The chief complaint for an established patient should be documented in Progress Notes unless a new history/physical examination form is being completed.

b. _____ When documenting the chief complaint in the medical record of an established patient, the same questions of when, where, how, and how long should be asked.

c. _____ After the physician identifies a diagnosis, it is permissible for the medical assistant to use that diagnosis in the documentation of the chief complaint.

d. _____ Proper spelling is not as important when documenting the care of an established patient since the physician has already spelled the medical terminology correctly in earlier Progress Notes.

e. _____ Documentation for an established patient is just as important as for a new patient.

f. _____ If the medical office has specific guidelines concerning documentation, these are not as important as those taught in class and should not be followed.

g. _____ When documenting in any medical record, the extern or medical assisting student should sign the medical record with the indication of student medical assistant (SMA).

h. _____ The medical assistant should document both objective and subjective symptoms in the medical record.

i. _____ If the physician has used a local abbreviation in the medical record, it is acceptable for the medical assistant to also use this abbreviation.

j. _____ Only clinical medical assistants document in medical records.

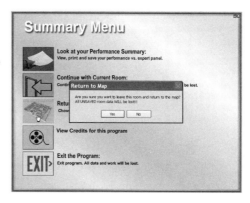

* Click **Close Chart** to return to the Exam Room.
* Click the exit arrow to leave the Exam Room.
* Select **Return to Map** from the Summary Menu.

Exercise 4

Online Activity—Documentation by Administrative Medical Assistants

 15 minutes

* From the patient list, select **Tristan Tsosie**.
  (*Note:* If you have exited the program, sign in
  again to Mountain View Clinic and select Tristan
  Tsosie from the patient list.)

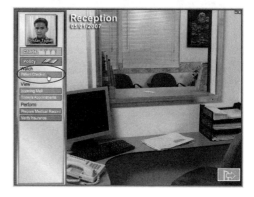

* On the office map, highlight and click on
  Reception to enter the check-in area.

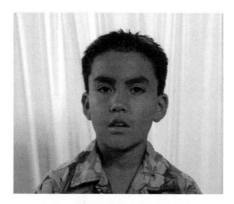

* Under the Watch heading, click on **Patient
  Check-In** to view the video.

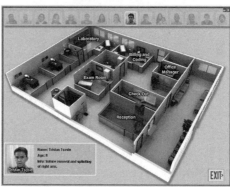

1. What important subjective symptoms does Tristan's sister report to the administrative medical assistant?

 • Click the exit arrow to leave the Reception desk.
 • Select **Return to Map** from the Summary Menu.
 • Keeping Tristan as your patient, highlight and click on **Check Out** on the office map.

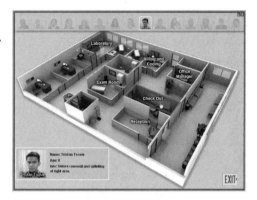

 • Next, click **Charts** and select **1-Progress Notes** from under the **Patient Medical Information** tab.
 • Read the initial documentation written by Dana Brick, CMA.

2. Which of the four questions that should be asked for accurate documentation of the chief complaint has been omitted from the Progress Notes, even though the sister provided the needed information when Tristan checked in?

3. Dana is a clinical medical assistant, and Kristin is an administrative medical assistant. Did the correct medical assistant document the information from the sister in the medical record?

4. How did you feel about the verbal and nonverbal communication between Kristin and Tristan and his sister during check-in? If you think there was a problem, how could it have been better handled?

• Click **Close Chart**; then click on the exit arrow.
 • Select **Return to Map** from the Summary Menu and continue to the next exercise.

Exercise 5

 Writing Activity—Practicing Documentation of History and Chief Complaint

 50 minutes

 • From the patient list, select **Wilson Metcalf**. (*Note:* If you have exited the program, sign in again to Mountain View Clinic and select Wilson Metcalf from the patient list.)

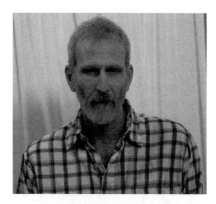

 • On the office map, highlight and click on **Check Out**.

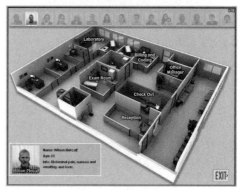

 • Click on **Charts** and then select **1-Progress Notes** from the drop-down menu under the **Patient Medical Information** tab.
 • Read the Progress Notes for Wilson Metcalf beginning with his initial visit to the office on 1/4/2007.

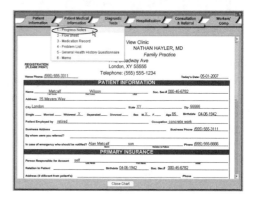

1. According to the Progress Notes, what were Mr. Metcalf's drinking habits at the time of his visit on 1/4/2007?

2. How much coffee did Mr. Metcalf admit to drinking in a day?

→ • Scroll down in the Progress Notes and read the documentation for the chief complaint for Mr. Metcalf's visit on 5/1/2007.

3. What are Mr. Metcalf's drinking habits now?

4. How much coffee does he currently admit to drinking in a day?

5. What was the diagnosis documented by Dr. Meyer on 1/4/2007?

6. What is Mr. Metcalf's diagnosis on 5/1/2007?

→ • Click on the **Patient Medical Information** tab again; this time, select **5-General Health History Questionnaire**.
• Click on the arrow at the top right corner of the screen to turn to page 2.
• Read Wilson Metcalf's Health History form that was completed on 1/4/2007.

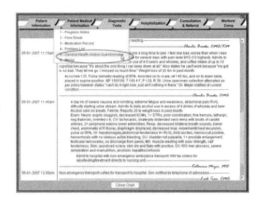

7. Who do you think filled out the Health History form?

8. Under Section IV, General Health Attitude and Habits, what was Mr. Metcalf's response to the question about how much alcohol he drinks, if any?

9. According to the form, did Mr. Metcalf believe he had a problem with alcohol?

10. On this form, how much coffee did Mr. Metcalf say he drank?

11. Are Wilson Metcalf's answers on the form consistent with the documentation in his Progress Notes? Explain. If the answers are not consistent, why do you think this may have happened?

12. Why would it have been important for the medical assistant to review this history with Wilson Metcalf?

13. Assume that you interviewed Wilson Metcalf on 1-4-2007 and wrote the Progress Notes on that date. Complete the blank page of the General Health History Questionnaire below by answering the questions correctly for Mr. Metcalf based on the information he provided during the interview.

Name   _Date_

Adult Health History Form

Your answers on this form will help your health care provider better understand your medical concerns and conditions better. This form will not be put directly into your medical chart. If you are uncomfortable with any question, do not answer it. If you cannot remember specific details, please provide your best guess. **Thank you!**

Age: _____   How would you rate your general health?   ❑ Excellent ❑ Good   ❑ Fair   ❑ Poor

Chief complaint: _____

Other concerns: _____

REVIEW OF SYMPTOMS: Please check any current symptoms you have.

Constitutional
_____ Recent fevers/sweats
_____ Unexplained weight loss/gain
_____ Unexplained fatigue/weakness

Ears/Nose/Throat/Mouth/Eyes
_____ Difficulty hearing/ringing in ears
_____ Hay fever/allergies/congestion
_____ Trouble swallowing
_____ Change in vision

Cardiovascular
_____ Chest pains/discomfort
_____ Palpitations
_____ Short of breath with exertion

Respiratory
_____ Cough/wheeze
_____ Coughing up blood

Gastrointestinal
_____ Heartburn/reflux
_____ Blood from rectum or change
        in bowel movement
_____ Nausea/vomitting/diarrhea
_____ Pain in abdomen

Neurological
_____ Headaches
_____ Memory loss
_____ Fainting

Musculoskeletal
_____ Muscle/joint pain
_____ Recent back pain

Blood/Lymphatic
_____ Unexplained lumps
_____ Easy bruising/bleeding

Genitourinary
_____ Painful/bloody urination
_____ Leaking urine
_____ Nighttime urination
_____ Discharge
_____ Concern with sexual functions

In the past month, have you had little interest or pleasure in doing things or felt down, depressed, or hopeless? ❑ Yes ❑ No

MEDICATIONS: Prescription and non-prescription medicines, vitamins, home remedies, herbs, etc.

Medication	Dose (e.g., mg/pill)	How many times per day

Allergies or reactions to medications: _____

PAST MEDICAL HISTORY: Please indicate whether you have had any of the following medical problems (with dates).

_____ Heart disease: _____ High blood pressure   _____ High cholesterol
    specify type: _____   _____ Diabetes   _____ Thyroid problem
_____ Asthma/Lung disease   _____ Other: (specify:) _____ _____ Kidney disease
                                                                      _____ Cancer: (specify): _____

SURGICAL HISTORY: Please list all prior operations (with dates): _____

FAMILY HISTORY: Please indicate the current status of your immediate family members.
Please indicate family members (parent, sibling, grandparent, aunt or uncle) with any of the following conditions:

Alcoholism _____   High cholesterol _____
Cancer, specify type _____   High blood pressure _____
Heart disease _____   Stroke _____
Depression/suicide _____   Bleeding or clotting disorder _____
Genetic disorders _____   Asthma/COPD _____
Diabetes _____   Other: _____

SOCIAL HISTORY:

Tobacco Use
Cigarettes ❑ Never ❑ Quit Date _____
  ❑ Current Smoker: packs/day _____ # of yrs _____
Other Tobacco: ❑ Pipe ❑ Cigar ❑ Snuff ❑ Chew
Are you interested in quitting?   ❑ No ❑ Yes

Alcohol Use
Do you drink alcohol?   ❑ No ❑ Yes # drinks/week ____
Is your alcohol use a concern for you or others?   ❑ No ❑ Yes

Drug Use
Do you use any recreational drugs?   ❑ No ❑ Yes
Have you ever used needles to inject drugs?   ❑ No ❑ Yes

Sexual Activity
Sexually active: ❑ No ❑ Yes ❑ Not currently

OTHER CONCERNS

Caffeine Intake: ❑ None ❑ Coffee/tea/soda _____ cups/day

Weight: Are you satisfied with your weight?   ❑ No ❑ Yes

Diet: How do you rate your diet?   ❑ Good ❑ Fair ❑ Poor
Do you eat or drink four servings of dairy or soy daily or take calcium supplements?   ❑ No ❑ Yes

Exercise: Do you exercise regularly?   ❑ No ❑ Yes
What kind of exercise? _____
How long (minutes) _____ How often? _____
If you do not exercise, why? _____

Safety:
Do you use seatbelts consistently?
Is violence at home a concern for you?   ❑ No ❑ Yes

Have you completed a living will or durable power of attorney for health care?   ❑ No ❑ Yes

SOCIOECONOMICS   Occupation: _____   Employer: _____
Years of education/highest degree: _____   Marital Status: Single Partner/Married Divorced Widowed Other: _____
Spouse/partner's name: _____   Number of chidren/ages: _____
Who lives at home with you? _____

14. Suppose that Mac Wallace (born 10-23-1980) comes to the office stating he has a fever and sore throat. He has had difficulty swallowing and has had pain in his right ear. All of these symptoms have lasted for about 4 days and have become progressively worse each day. He has also run out of blood pressure medicine and wants the prescription to be refilled. Before his throat became sore, his child had strep throat. Document Mac Wallace's chief complaint on the Progress Notes below.

PATIENT'S NAME		☐ FEMALE ☐ MALE Date of Birth: __/__/__
DATE	**PATIENT VISITS AND FINDINGS**	

ALLERGIC TO _____

_____ PAGE _____ of _____

15. What subjective symptoms does Mac Wallace report?

Obtaining Vital Signs

👓 **Reading Assignment:** Chapter 31—Vital Signs
- • Factors That May Influence Vital Signs
- • Temperature
- • Pulse
- • Respiration
- • Blood Pressure

Patients: Teresa Hernandez, John R. Simmons

Learning Objectives:

- State the normal range for body temperature, based on the site used to measure the reading.
- Identify conditions that alter body temperature.
- State the normal range for pulse rate.
- Identify the three terms used to describe pulse rate and rhythm.
- Describe conditions that alter pulse rate and rhythm.
- Identify terms related to vital signs.
- State the normal respiratory rate, depth, and rhythm.
- Describe conditions that alter respiratory function.
- State the normal ranges for blood pressure.
- Describe conditions that alter body pressure, including age-related factors.
- Discuss what is meant by hypertension, prehypertension, and normal blood pressure.

Overview:

This lesson is intended to provide an understanding of the importance of obtaining vital signs correctly. Dr. John R. Simmons is a college professor who has a history of hypertension. Teresa Hernandez is a teenage patient. You will be using the Policy Manual to decide what steps you need to include in patient care to be in compliance with the physician's standing orders for these patients.

Exercise 1

Online Activity—Obtaining Temperature, Pulse, and Respiration

60 minutes

- Sign in to Mountain View Clinic.
- From the patient list, select **Teresa Hernandez**.

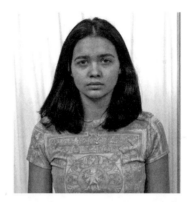

- On the office map, highlight and click on **Exam Room**.

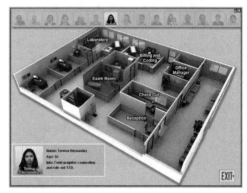

- Select **Policy** to open the office Policy Manual.
- Type "standing orders" in the search bar and click the magnifying glass twice to read the relevant section.
- When finished, click **Close Manual** to return to the Exam Room.
- Answer the following questions regarding documentation of vital signs.

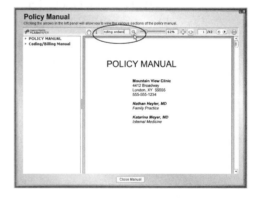

1. What are the standing order instructions regarding vital signs and physical examinations?

2. List five factors that can affect body temperature.

   (1)

   (2)

   (3)

   (4)

   (5)

3. If you were to check the temperature of a 6-year-old child who was playing outside in the sun during summer, would you expect the child's temperature to be slightly elevated?

4. What course of action could you take to double-check and ensure that the body temperature was higher as a result of activity rather than illness?

5. A person with fever is described as _____, whereas a person without

   fever is considered _____.

6. Which of the following temperature readings would be considered normal in an adult patient?
   a. Oral 98.6
   b. Axillary 97.6
   c. Tympanic 98.6
   d. All of the above

7. Below, match each normal temperature with the age group to which it applies.

Age Group	Normal Temperature
_____ Newborn	a. 98.6 oral
_____ 1 year	b. 96.8 oral
_____ 6 years to adult	c. 98.2 axillary
_____ Elderly, over age 70 years	d. 99.7

8. What is specifically being measured when a person's pulse rate is obtained?

9. Consider all the patients at Mountain View Clinic. Which patient would you expect to have the highest pulse rate, as determined by age only?

10. List the most common pulse sites.

11. Match each of the following age groups with the average pulse rate that applies.

Average Pulse Rate	Age Group
_____ 75-120	a. Newborns
_____ 60-100	b. 1-2 years
_____ 80-140	c. 3-6 years
_____ 120-160	d. 7-11 years
_____ 75-110	e. Adolescence to adulthood

12. Three characteristics of the patient's pulse are described by the terms

_____, _____, and _____.

13. What is meant by dysrhythmia?

14. When discussing pulse volume, _____ indicates a fast, weak pulse,

    whereas _____ indicates an extremely full pulse.

15. The number of breaths (full inspiration and full expiration) that a patient takes during a

    60-second interval should be documented as the patient's respiratory _____.

16. Which of the following factors affect respirations? Select all that apply.

    _____ Age

    _____ Exercise

    _____ Environment

    _____ Disease processes

    _____ Emotional states

    _____ Gender

    _____ Medications

17. Match each of the following respiratory terms to its definition.

Term	**Definition**
_____ Rhonchi	a. A condition marked by rapid shallow respiration
_____ Wheezes	b. Abnormally prolonged and deep breathing associated with acute anxiety or emotional
_____ Hyperventilation	tension
_____ Tachypnea	c. Abnormal rumbling sounds on expiration that indicate airway obstruction by thick secretions or spasms
	d. High-pitched sound heard on expiration that indicates an obstruction or narrowing of the respiratory passages

18. Match each of the following average respiratory rate ranges with the age group to which it applies.

Average Respiratory Rate Range	**Age Group**
_____ 12-20	a. Newborns
_____ 20-30	b. 1-3 years
_____ 30-50	c. 4-6 years
_____ 16-22	d. 7-11 years
_____ 18-26	e. Adolescents/adults

19. The taking in of oxygen is called _____, whereas the breathing out of carbon dioxide is called _____. Together, these two mechanisms are considered one _____.

20. Match each of the following terms with its definition.

Definition	**Term**
_____ Dyspnea that is relieved by standing or sitting positions	a. Apnea
_____ Bluish discoloration of the skin	b. Sleep apnea
_____ Difficult breathing	c. Stertorous
_____ Absence of respiration	d. Orthopnea
_____ Strenuous respiratory effort marked by a snoring sound	e. Dyspnea
_____ Absence of respirations during periods of rest	f. Cyanosis

21. Indicate whether each of the following statements is true or false.

a. _____ When an aural temperature is taken on a toddler, the auricle should be pulled down and back.

b. _____ When an aural temperature is taken on an adult, the auricle should be pulled up and back to expose the tympanic membrane.

c. _____ The patient should be told what procedures will be done when obtaining all vital signs.

d. _____ If a pulse rate is being taken prior to counting the respiratory rate, you should count the respiratory rate after releasing the pressure from the patient's wrist.

e. _____ Measuring a rectal temperature is a safe procedure for all patients.

f. _____ All patients can have the pulse taken at the radial site.

g. _____ When pulse rates are being recorded, any deviation of rhythm or volume should be documented.

h. _____ When respirations are being recorded, any deviation in rhythm or volume should be documented.

Now that you have reviewed information regarding taking vital signs, continue with Teresa Hernandez as your patient.

- From the Exam Room menu, click on **Take Vital Signs** (under the Perform heading).
- As you click on each vital sign, the reading will appear in the corresponding box. Note there is a check box to mark if the physician needs to be notified of any abnormality. At the bottom of the screen there is room for you to document each vital sign for the patient.

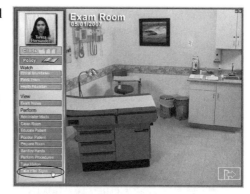

- Record the readings accurately and click **Finish** to return to the **Exam Room**. You may exit and go to **Look at Your Performance Summary**. Scroll down and check your answers with the experts.

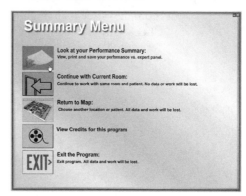

22. Which, if any, of Teresa Hernandez's vital signs are not within normal limits?

23. If Teresa's pulse rate had been 148, would you have needed to alert the physician?

24. Suppose Teresa has just arrived at the office when you call her name and take her to the examination room. When you take her vital signs, her pulse is 148 and her respiratory rate is 36. While you are recording her chief complaint, Teresa mentions she is out of breath because the elevator was out of order and she had to walk up 16 flights of stairs to make it to the appointment. Does this have any bearing on the readings you obtained? If yes, why?

25. What would be an appropriate thing to do in this instance?

 • Select **Return to Map** from the Summary Menu.
• From the office map, highlight and click on **Check Out** to review the final documentation of Teresa's visit.

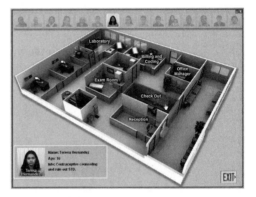

• Open **Charts** and select **1-Progress Notes** from the drop-down menu under the **Patient Medical Information** tab.
• Read the entire documentation of Teresa Hernandez's visit for this date.
• Click **Close Chart** to return to the Check Out desk.
• On the Summary Menu, click **Return to Map**.

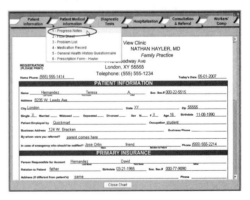

26. Did the medical assistant obtain the necessary vital signs? Explain your answer.

Exercise 2

Online Activity—Obtaining Blood Pressure Readings

45 minutes

Before you sign in to Mountain View Clinic, answer the following questions about measuring and recording blood pressure.

1. What is specifically assessed by blood pressure measurements?

2. The top number of the blood pressure reading is referred to as the _____

   reading, and the bottom number is referred to as the _____ reading.

3. Match each of the following terms with its definition.

Term	Definition
_____ Hypertension	a. Pressure on the walls of the arteries when the heart is relaxed and the last sound is heard
_____ Pulse pressure	b. Blood pressure over 140/90
_____ Systolic pressure	c. Blood pressure below 90/50
_____ Hypotension	d. Highest pressure that occurs when the heart is contracting and the first pulse beat is heard
_____ Diastolic pressure	e. The difference between systolic and diastolic pressure

4. Which of the following factors affect blood pressure? Select all that apply.

    _____ Time of day

    _____ Age

    _____ Environment

    _____ Exercise

    _____ Gender

    _____ Emotions

    _____ Body position

    _____ Amount of sleep

    _____ Medications

5. List the numerical categories for defining normal blood pressure, prehypertensive state, and hypertension, as published by the American Heart Association.

6. List nine symptoms that patients may experience that could be caused by undiagnosed hypertension.

7. The equipment needed for obtaining blood pressure includes a _____

    and _____.

8. If John R. Simmons were the patient, which size blood pressure cuff would you need to choose to check his blood pressure?

9. If Tristan Tsosie were the patient, which size blood pressure cuff would you need to choose to check his blood pressure?

10. The sounds heard through the stethoscope as the blood pressure is being taken are called

_____.

- From the patient list, select **John R. Simmons**. The overview states that Dr. John Simmons is a professor. (*Note:* If you have exited the program, sign in again to Mountain View Clinic and select John R. Simmons from the patient list.)
- On the office map, click **Reception** and watch the video.

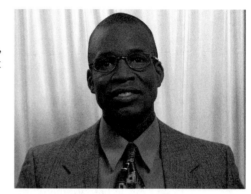

Critical Thinking Question

11. How should the office staff address John Simmons?

- On the office map, click on **Check Out**.

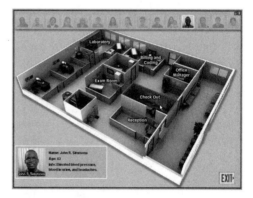

- Click on **Charts** and select **1-Progress Notes** from the drop-down menu under the **Patient Medical Information** tab.
- Read the entire documentation of Dr. Simmons' visit.

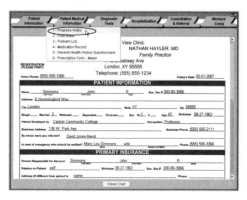

12. Dr. Simmons had his blood pressure monitored throughout his visit. Which, if any, of the vital signs for Dr. Simmons are not within normal limits?

13. The blood pressure readings for Dr. Simmons are higher when taken the second time. What is a logical explanation for the difference?

14. Why do you think that Dr. Meyer wants Dr. Simmons to take blood pressure readings at home and record them?

15. Notice that Dr. Simmons' blood pressure reading taken from the left arm is more elevated than the reading from the right arm. What is an explanation for this?

Exercise 3

Writing Activity—Documentation of Vital Signs

10 minutes

1. Using today's date and time, accurately document the following scenario on the form below:

   Judy Marks, age 69 years (born 4-27-38), is taking medication for hypertensive disease and is seen at the office on a regular basis. Today she has come in to have her vital signs checked by the medical assistant. Her pulse is 104, weak, and difficult to obtain, with a skipped beat every six beats. Her rate of breathing is 24 times a minute but shallow. Her temperature is 97.6 degrees. Her blood pressure is 176/104 in the left arm and 170/102 in the right arm.

PATIENT'S NAME _____   ☐ FEMALE   ☐ MALE   Date of Birth: __ / __ / __

DATE	PATIENT VISITS AND FINDINGS

ALLERGIC TO _____

_____ PAGE_____ of _____

2. Which, if any, of the findings on the form in the previous question need to be reported to the physician before Judy Marks leaves the office? Which are abnormal?

Measuring Height and Weight

∽◯刃 **Reading Assignment:** Chapter 31—Vital Signs
  • Anthropometric Measurement

Patients: Shaunti Begay, Jean Deere

Learning Objectives:

• Describe the correct methodology for measuring height on an adult.
• Describe the correct methodology for measuring weight on an adult.
• Convert height from inches to feet and inches.
• Convert height and weight from metric to English measurements.
• Convert height and weight from English to metric measurements.
• State the importance of measuring height and weight on each office visit.

Overview:

In this lesson you will describe the correct methodology for measuring height and weight on a teenager and an adult. You will demonstrate how to convert a patient's height from inches to feet and inches for documentation. You will also perform conversions between metric and English measurements. One of the patients, Jean Deere, is confused. You will observe the handling of this patient and critique the actions of the medical assistant.

Exercise 1

Online Activity—Measuring Height

🕐 30 minutes

- Sign in to Mountain View Clinic.
- From the patient list, select **Shaunti Begay**.

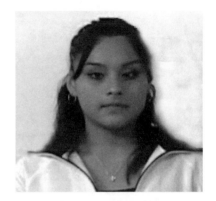

- On the office map, highlight and click on **Exam Room**.

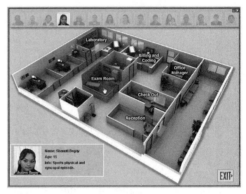

- Under the Watch heading, select **Health Promotion** to view the video.

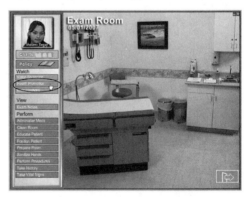

- Using the control buttons at the bottom of the video screen, stop the video at the first fade-out.

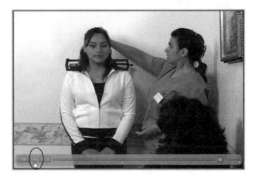

- Click **Close** to return to the Exam Room.

1. Why should Shaunti remove her shoes before her height and weight are measured?

2. Why is it important to measure a child's height at each office visit through adolescence?

3. What may occur in regard to height as an adult person ages?

4. Shaunti is wearing socks. If she were not wearing socks, what would have been the appropriate action by the medical assistant before having her stand on the scale?

5. What is the correct angle of the head bar when measuring height?

6. The height measurements on medical scales are marked in _____-inch increments.

7. The medical assistant stated that Shaunti is 5 feet 2 inches tall, which would be _____ inches.

8. How do you think Shaunti felt about her mother's comment in regard to her weight?

 • Click the exit arrow at the bottom right of the screen to leave the Exam Room.
• From the Summary Menu, click **Return to Map**.

Exercise 2

 Online Activity—Measuring Weight

 30 minutes

1. How is quality control performed on scales?

2. What safety steps does the medical assistant need to take with all patients when measuring weight?

3. What weight calibration marking is used on most standing scales found in medical offices?

 • From the patient list, select **Jean Deere**. (*Note:* If you have exited the program, sign in again to Mountain View Clinic and select Jean Deere from the patient list.)

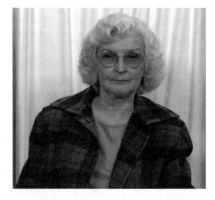

• On the office map, highlight and click on **Exam Room**.

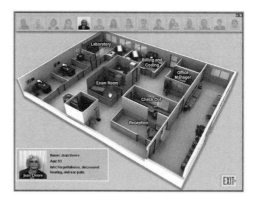

• Under the Watch heading, select **Patient Assessment** to view the video.
• At the end of the video, click **Close** to return to the Exam Room.

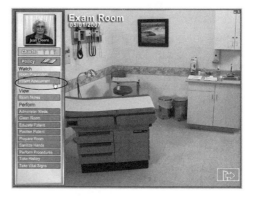

4. Did the medical assistant handle Ms. Deere appropriately to obtain an accurate measurement of the patient's weight?

5. The medical assistant offered to help Ms. Deere to the scales. Why would this be so important with this patient?

6. Notice the placement of the walker over the scales. Why is this important to help in supporting Ms. Deere? When a walker is used in this way, what observations must the medical assistant make to ensure an accurate reading?

7. Ms. Deere is confused, and her son thinks she might have early Alzheimer's disease. Do you think that the medical assistant was professional and appropriate in her handling of the patient? Explain your answer. Was it appropriate for Ms. Deere's son to be with her during the weight measurement? Why or why not?

→ • In the Exam Room, click on **Charts** and select **1-Progress Notes** from the drop-down menu under the **Patient Medical Information** tab.

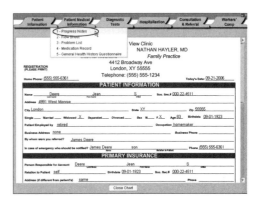

8. Based on the Progress Notes, what was Jean Deere's weight on her last visit on 9/21/06?

9. Ms. Deere's weight on this visit is 120 pounds. Do you see a reason for the medical assistant to ask questions about her eating habits while taking the health history? Explain.

→ • Click **Close Chart** to return to the Exam Room.
  • Click on **Policy** to open the office Policy Manual.
  • In the search bar, type "standing orders" and click twice on the magnifying glass to read the relevant section of the manual.

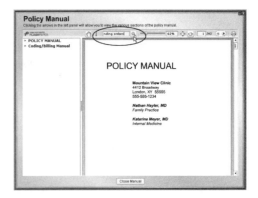

10. Did the medical assistants follow the correct protocol for Shaunti Begay and Jean Deere, according to what you read in the Policy Manual? Explain your answer.

Critical Thinking Question

11. If a patient tells the medical assistant that he or she prefers not to be weighed, but it is the protocol of the office that all patients be weighed, what would be the best way for the medical assistant to proceed?

Exercise 3

Writing Activity—Conversions for Mensuration

15 minutes

Use the formulas provided below to calculate answers to the questions in this exercise.

- Weight conversion of kilograms to pounds: Multiply kilograms by 2.2 (1 kg = 2.2 lb).
- Weight conversion of pounds to kilograms: Divide kilograms by 2.2 (2.2 lb = 1 kg).
- Height conversion of inches to feet and inches: Divide the total number of inches by 12; then express the remainder as inches (12 in = 1 ft).
- Height conversion of inches to centimeters: Multiply inches by 2.5 (1 in = 2.5 cm).
- Height conversion of centimeters to inches: Divide centimeters by 2.5 (2.5 cm = 1 in).

1. Joan Neiman weighs 64 kilograms. What is her weight in pounds?

2. Shaunti Begay is 5 feet 2 inches tall. What is her height in centimeters?

3. Jean Deere weighs 120 pounds. What is her weight in kilograms?

4. Sara McHugh is 68 inches tall. What is her height in feet and inches?

5. Isaiah Franklin is 185 centimeters tall. What is his height in inches? In feet and inches?

Preparing and Maintaining Examination and Treatment Areas

Reading Assignment: Chapter 32—Assisting with the Primary Physical Examination
- Physical Examination
- Preparing for the Physical Examination
- Supplies and Instruments Needed for the Physical Examination

Patients: Jean Deere, Louise Parlet, Rhea Davison, Jesus Santo

Learning Objectives:

- Describe the steps necessary in preparing an examination room for patient care.
- List supplies needed for a complete physical examination.
- Describe the steps necessary in cleaning the examination or treatment room following patient care.

Overview:

In this lesson you will list the supplies that are necessary in preparing an examination or treatment room for patient Jean Deere. After the patient has been examined by the physician, the examination/treatment room must be prepared for the next patient, Louise Parlet. Finally, a review of the necessary steps in infection control and disposal of biohazardous waste will be presented, including questions addressing correct hand hygiene.

Exercise 1

Online Activity—Preparing the Examination or Treatment Room for Patient Care

30 minutes

- Sign in to Mountain View Clinic.
- From the patient list, select **Jean Deere**.

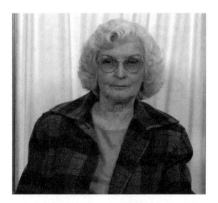

- On the office map, highlight and click on **Exam Room**.

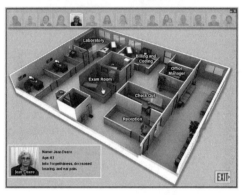

- Click on **Policy** to open the office Policy Manual.

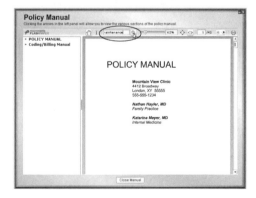

- In the search bar type "room maintenance" and click once on the magnifying glass. Read the office policy for the preparation of exam/treatment rooms.

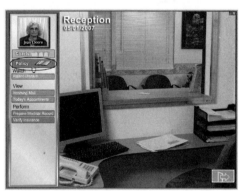

- Click **Close Manual** to return to the Exam Room.
- Under the Watch heading, select **Room Preparation** to review the video on room preparation.
- At the end of the video, click **Close** to return to the Exam Room.

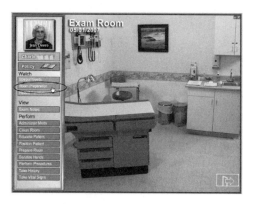

1. The medical assisting extern washed her hands before setting up the exam/treatment room. Why is this an important step in room preparation?

2. The medical assistant extern asked Ameeta about Ms. Deere's symptoms. Why is this information important when preparing a room for the patient?

3. Indicate whether each of the following statements is true or false.

   a. _____ Infection control is important when preparing a room for a patient.

   b. _____ When preparing the room for a physical examination, all equipment must be in good working order, properly disinfected, and readily available for the physician's use during the examination.

   c. _____ The general cleanliness of the room has nothing to do with the patient's feelings about the entire medical office.

   d. _____ Waste receptacles in the examination/treatment room should be emptied frequently.

   e. _____ Biohazardous receptacles should be changed after any patient care that involves gross biohazard waste.

   f. _____ Sharps biohazard containers should be emptied daily.

g. _____ Equipment for the examination should be placed at easy access for the physician and, if possible, in the order of use.

h. _____ The medical assistant should know how to operate and care for the equipment found in examination and treatment rooms.

i. _____ The appropriate room temperature should be determined by what is comfortable for the physician.

j. _____ All equipment in the exam room should be disposable.

k. _____ Proper disposal of equipment following use is an important factor in infection control.

l. _____ Improperly checked equipment and supplies may cause injury to a patient.

4. Match each of the following pieces of equipment to its description or purpose.

Equipment	**Description or Purpose**
_____ Sphygmomanometer	a. Light on a movable stand
_____ Drape	b. Covering to reduce patient exposure
_____ Patient gown	c. Used to test neurological reflexes
_____ Thermometer	d. Long stick with cotton cover used to obtain specimens or to cleanse an area when dampened
_____ Cotton-tipped applicator	e. Small flashlight used to check the pupils
_____ Tongue depressor	f. Instrument used to check hearing
_____ Lubricant	g. Instrument used to measure blood pressure
_____ Tape measure	h. Instrument used to measure temperature
_____ Tuning fork	i. Instrument used to auscultate sounds
_____ Percussion hammer	j. A device used to measure parts of the body
_____ Speculum	k. A covering for hands for good infection control practices
_____ Ophthalmoscope	l. A covering with sleeves to provide modesty and warmth for the patient
_____ Otoscope	m. Smooth wooden blade used to examine the mouth and throat
_____ Stethoscope	n. Instrument used to examine the eyes
_____ Penlight	o. Instrument used to open a body orifice
_____ Gooseneck lamp	p. Instrument used to examine the ear canal
_____ Disposable gloves	q. Agent used to reduce friction

➡ • Click on **Exam Notes** to open the physician's notes about Ms. Deere for this visit. When finished reading, click **Finish** to return to the Exam Room.

5. Ameeta was correct in assuming Dr. Meyer would want to do an ear lavage and a pulse oximeter reading. What additional test did Dr. Meyer want done at this visit?

➡ • Under the Perform heading, select **Prepare Room**.

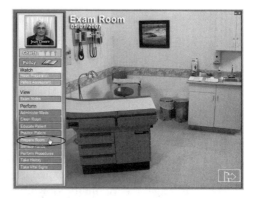

• Select the first item needed for Ms. Deere's visit from the Available Supplies list and click **Add Item** to confirm your choice. The items you select will appear in the Selected Supplies box.

• Repeat this step until you are satisfied you have everything you need from the list. (*Note:* The Exam Notes are available if you need to refer to them.)

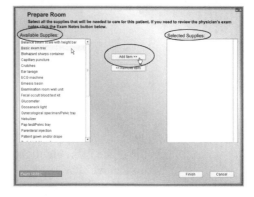

• After making all your selections, click **Finish** to return to the Exam Room.

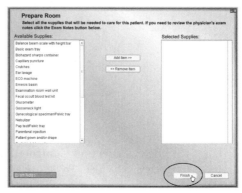

• Click the exit arrow to go to the Summary Menu.

• Click on **Look at Your Performance Summary**. Scroll down to the Prepare Room section to compare your answers with those of the experts. This summary can also be printed or saved for your instructor.

• Click on **Close** to return to the Summary Menu.

• Click on **Return to Map** and continue to the next exercise.

6. What impact would the things you initially left off the list have on patient care?

Exercise 2

Online Activity—Maintaining the Examination or Treatment Room Following Patient Care

 30 minutes

- From the patient list, select **Louise Parlet**. (*Note:* If you have exited the program, sign in again to Mountain View Clinic and select Louise Parlet from the patient list.)

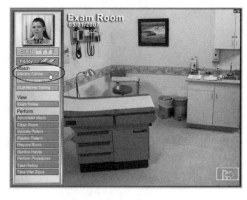

- On the office map, highlight and click on the **Exam Room**.

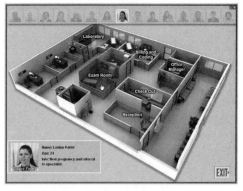

- Select **Infection Control** (under Watch) and view the video. Pay close attention to the extern's actions throughout the entire video. At the end of the video, click **Close** to return to the Exam Room.

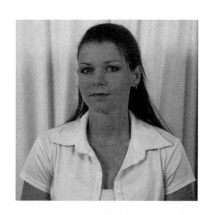

- Next, click on **Policy** to open the Policy Manual.
- In the search bar, type "room maintenance" and click on the magnifying glass to review.

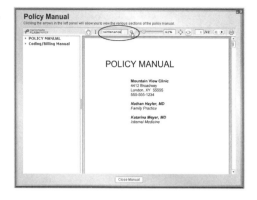

1. What does the Policy Manual indicate should be performed after each patient has been seen?

2. During the video, did the medical assistant follow the Policy Manual while cleaning the room? Explain your answer.

3. During the video, did you see a break in infection control by the medical assisting extern? Explain.

4. Would it have been acceptable for the medical assisting extern to clean the table without gloves if she had sanitized her hands prior to and immediately after disposing of the table paper and gown? Why or why not?

5. After the extern has cleaned the examination table and removed her gloves, what is the appropriate means of hand hygiene?

6. Indicate whether each of the following statements is true or false.

a. _____ The medical assistant should use gloves, gown, and face shield when cleaning the exam room after a patient.

b. _____ The medical assistant should disinfect the table, supply tray, and counter/table tops after each patient.

c. _____ The nondisposable supplies and equipment should be disinfected and properly stored when cleaning the room.

d. _____ Nondisposable equipment should be sanitized and sterilized as necessary before storage.

e. _____ The office Policy Manual contains all information needed for the correct cleaning of a room following any type of patient examination.

f. _____ The physician will inform the medical assistant of the items that must be discarded and those that should be sanitized and used again.

g. _____ Items such as ophthalmoscopes, otoscopes, and tuning forks do not require sanitization following use in patient care.

h. _____ Standard precautions should be followed when preparing and cleaning the examination/treatment room.

i. _____ If the medical assistant does not have time between patients to completely clean the room, it is more important to keep the appointment schedule on time than to clean the room.

j. _____ It is permissible for the medical assistant to clean a room after the following patient has been placed in the examination/treatment room.

k. _____ Teamwork is essential in keeping the office neat, clean, and ready for patients.

7. What do you think would be the best action to take if you enter a room with a patient and discover that the room has not been prepared as it should be?

Exercise 3

 Online Activity—Maintaining and Cleaning the Treatment Room Following Patient Care

 10 minutes

• From the patient list, select **Rhea Davison**. (*Note:* If you have exited the program, sign in again to Mountain View Clinic and select Rhea Davison from the patient list.)

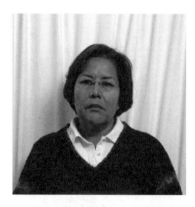

• On the office map, highlight and click on the **Exam Room**.

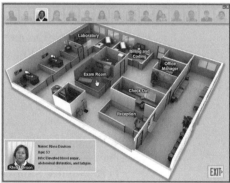

- Under View, select **Exam Notes** and review the patient's notes. To exit, click **Finish**.
- Select **Clean Room** (under Perform) and choose the appropriate things to do to correctly clean the room after Rhea Davison's examination. After making your selections, click **Finish**.
- Next, click on the exit arrow and select **Look at Your Performance Summary** to compare your choices with those of the experts.
- Click **Close** and then select **Return to Map**.

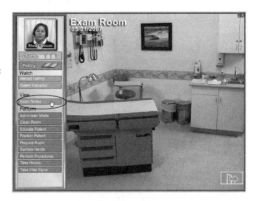

- From the patient list, select **Jesus Santo**.

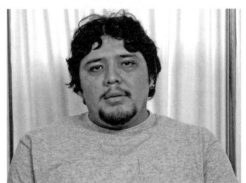

- On the office map, highlight and click on the **Exam Room**.

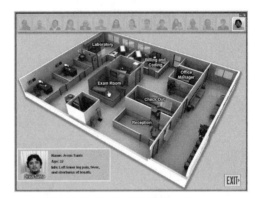

- Under View, select **Exam Notes** and review the patient's notes. Click **Finish** when you are done reviewing.
- Select **Clean Room** (under Perform) and choose the appropriate things to do to correctly clean the room after Jesus Santo's examination. After making your selections, click **Finish**.
- Next, click on the exit arrow and select **Look at Your Performance Summary** to compare your results with those of the experts.

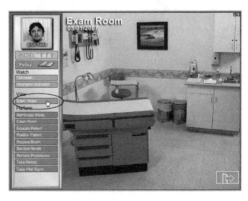

Preparing the Patient and Assisting with a Routine Physical Examination

LESSON 18

Reading Assignment: Chapter 32—Assisting with the Primary Physical Examination
- Physical Examination
- Assisting with the Physical Examination
- Principles of Body Mechanics
- Examination Sequence
- Role of the Medical Assistant

Patients: Teresa Hernandez, Jean Deere

Learning Objectives:

- Identify the information needed to prepare the patient for a physical examination.
- Prepare the patient for a physical examination following office policy and procedures.
- Understand legal and ethical boundaries when preparing a patient for a physical examination.
- Choose the correct patient positioning for the physical examination.
- Recognize the ethical role of the medical assistant when assisting with a physical examination.
- Discuss patient safety measures during a physical examination.
- Describe the importance of time efficiency when assisting the examiner.
- Understand the importance of using correct body mechanics while assisting with physical examinations.
- Recognize what instruments are needed when assisting with the physical examination.

Overview:

In this lesson you will study the necessary steps in patient preparation for a routine physical examination. Teresa Hernandez is a new teenage patient, whereas Jean Deere is an established geriatric patient. Ms. Deere wants her son James to assist in getting her ready for a physical examination. With each patient, ethical and legal issues are of concern.

Exercise 1

Online Activity—Preparing an Established Patient for Physical Examination

 20 minutes

- Sign in to Mountain View Clinic.
- From the patient list, select **Jean Deere**.

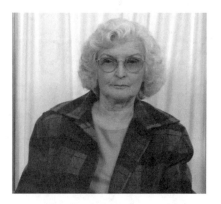

- On the office map, highlight and click on **Exam Room**.

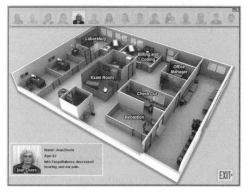

- Under the Watch heading, select **Patient Assessment** to view the video.
- At the end of the video, click **Close** to return to the Exam Room.

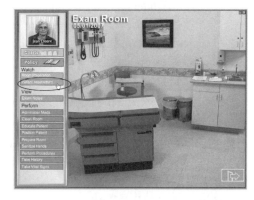

- Click on **Policy** to open the office Policy Manual. Type "standing orders" in the search bar.
- Click twice on the magnifying glass and read the Standing Orders section (pages 23-26).
- Click **Close Manual** to return to the Exam Room.

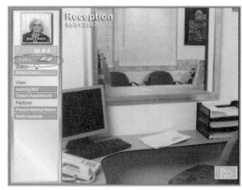

1. What clothing should be removed for Ms. Deere's physical examination?

2. What supplies should Ameeta be sure are available on the table to assist Ms. Deere's son James in preparing his mother for the examination?

3. Ameeta has allowed Ms. Deere's son to assist with disrobing. Is that appropriate? Why or why not?

4. When would it not be appropriate to allow a family member to help disrobe a patient?

5. Why is it important for Ameeta to offer to help Ms. Deere onto the table?

6. If Ms. Deere seemed to be weak on her left side, to which side would Ameeta provide support, while using the correct body mechanics?

7. For safety reasons, when should Ms. Deere be positioned on the examination table?

8. Is it acceptable to leave the room when a confused, debilitated, or geriatric patient is on the examination table? Why or why not?

9. What position would be appropriate for placing Ms. Deere on the examination table?

→ • Click the exit arrow to leave the Exam Room.
   • From the Summary Menu, click on **Return to Map** and continue to the next exercise.

Exercise 2

 Online Activity—Preparing a Young Adult and Assisting with a Routine Physical Examination

 25 minutes

- From the patient list, select **Teresa Hernandez**. (*Note:* If you have exited the program, sign in again to Mountain View Clinic and select Teresa Hernandez from the patient list.)

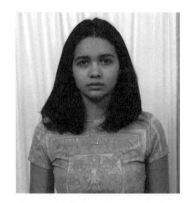

- On the office map, highlight and click on **Reception**.

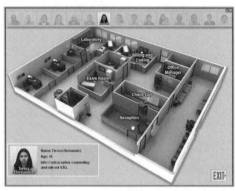

- Click on **Today's Appointments** to view the schedule. On the schedule find the reason for Teresa Hernandez's visit.

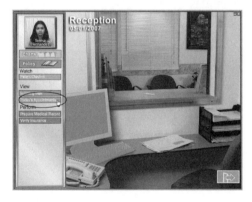

- Click **Finish** to close the appointment book and return to the Reception desk.

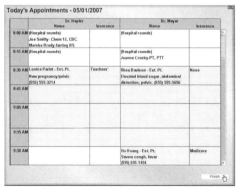

- Click on **Patient Check-In** to view the video.
- If you wish, you may also review the Policy Manual section on Standing Orders once more before answering the following questions.

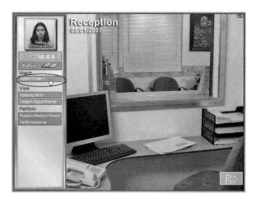

1. What is the reason for Teresa Hernandez's appointment, and what is her status in the medical office that will affect preparations for the physical examination?

2. Did you feel that Kristin was professional in speaking with Teresa about correcting the forms she was asked to fill out, even though Teresa was concerned about her parents finding out she had an appointment at the office?

- Click on the exit arrow to leave Reception.
- From the Summary Menu, click **Return to Map**.
- On the office map, highlight and click on **Exam Room**.

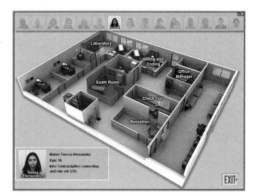

• Select **Ethical Boundaries** (under Watch) to view the video. At the end of the video, click **Close** to return to the Exam Room.

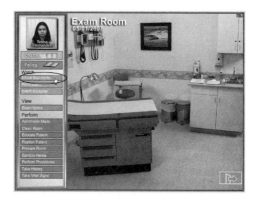

3. What preliminary steps must the clinical medical assistant complete before a physical examination?

4. What clothing should Teresa remove for her physical examination?

5. Teresa appears to be very nervous and uneasy about discussing her chief complaint. What do you think of the way that Ameeta, the medical assistant, handled the situation?

6. Because of the privacy issues surrounding contraception, especially with a teenage patient, Ameeta was faced with ethical and confidentiality boundaries in preparing Teresa to talk with the physician. Do you think that Ameeta provided the guidance needed to place Teresa more at ease? Explain your answer.

7. Would it have been appropriate for Ameeta to tell Teresa that what is said in the office is confidential? Why or why not?

8. Ameeta instructed Teresa to completely disrobe and to put on the gown, but can you identify any important information that she did not include in her instructions?

→ • Under Watch, select and view the next video, **Pelvic Examination**.

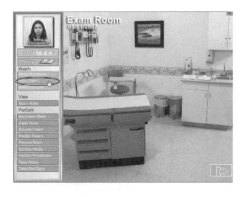

9. In the video, what are the ways that Ameeta assists Dr. Hayler? Select all that apply.

_____ Passes instruments

_____ Takes instruments after use

_____ Waits for Dr. Hayler to ask for instruments

_____ Is prepared to give Dr. Hayler the needed supplies promptly

_____ Explains the procedure and the need for infection control

_____ Disposes of Dr. Hayler's disposable equipment

_____ Asks Dr. Hayler to dispose of the equipment

_____ Has prepared the tray and passes all supplies on the tray for use

_____ Has the supplies prepared that might be used for a pelvic examination

_____ Accepts specimen for laboratory testing

_____ Prepares a label for specimen transport

_____ Has gooseneck lamp adjusted for proper lighting of area being examined

_____ Has the patient in the proper position for a pelvic examination

10. How did Ameeta provide safety measures for Teresa?

11. What was one thing Ameeta could have asked Teresa to do before helping her sit up.

12. Why is it important for Ameeta to have all the supplies and equipment available for the physician and to efficiently hand these to the physician without the physician having to ask?

13. Teresa was placed in the _____ position.

Exercise 3

Writing Activity—Appropriate Body Mechanics

10 minutes

Answer the following questions regarding using proper body mechanics while assisting with patient examinations.

1. If you are reaching for an object, you should avoid twisting and turning and instead move your feet to face the object. What is the purpose of doing this?

2. What is the risk involved with placing the popliteal area of your legs behind the knees next to the edge of the chair?

3. It is advisable to not cross your legs while sitting. What is the reason for this recommendation?

4. What precautions should be taken when lifting heavy objects?

Administering Parenteral Medications and Immunizations

Reading Assignment: Chapter 33—Principles of Pharmacology
- Drug Names
- Factors That Affect Drug Action

Chapter 34—Pharmacology Math

Chapter 35—Administering Medications
- Safety in Drug Administration
- Drug Forms and Administration

Patients: Shaunti Begay, Jesus Santo, Jade Wong

Learning Objectives:

- Identify the correct dose (volume) of medication for a patient using the physician's order.
- Discuss the steps necessary to administer a parenteral injection according to the physician's orders.
- Choose appropriate supplies for assisting with the administration of medication (based on volume ordered).
- Identify the correct supplies for assisting with an examination.
- List the seven "Rights" of patient medication administration.
- Identify the necessary steps for patient safety with the administration of medications.
- Identify local resources for immunizations and for patient education.
- Correlate the importance of timing the collection of laboratory specimens with the administration of medication.
- Choose the appropriate biohazard container for disposal of supplies utilized in the administration of medication.
- Understand documentation and recordkeeping procedures for the administration of medication and immunizations.
- Correctly document the administration of medication.

Overview:

In this lesson the administration of medication based on the physician's order is presented. You will choose syringes and the volume of medication to help prepare patients for the administration of parenteral medications and immunizations. You will also complete the documentation of these injections. The appropriate way to provide referrals to community resources for health maintenance and prevention will also be presented.

217

Exercise 1

Online Activity—Administering Parenteral Medications

20 minutes

- Sign in to Mountain View Clinic.
- From the patient list, select **Jesus Santo**.

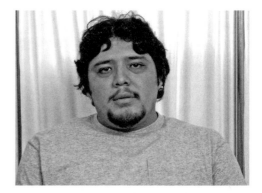

- On the office map, highlight and click on **Exam Room**.

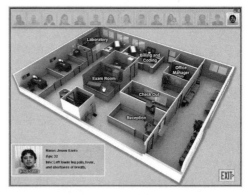

- Click on **Exam Notes** (under View) and read the documentation on Mr. Santo's visit for today.

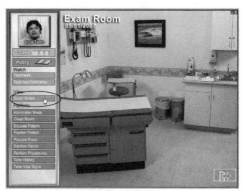

- Click **Finish** to return to the Exam Room.
- Under the Perform heading, click on **Prepare Room** to select the supplies needed for Mr. Santo's visit. (*Note:* You can reopen the Exam Notes for reference as you make your selections.)

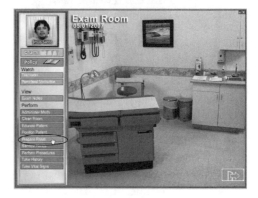

- Select the first item needed for Mr. Santo's visit from the alphabetical list and click **Add Item** to confirm your choice. The items you select will appear in the Selected Supplies column.
- Repeat this step until you are satisfied you have everything you need from the list.
- Do NOT close this window. Keep the Prepare Room wizard open as you continue with the lesson.

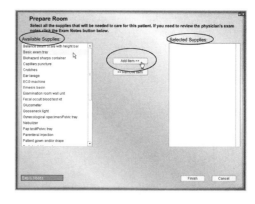

1. The medical assistant is asked to prepare Bicillin-LA 1,200,000 units for injection. If the medication is available as Bicillin-LA 600,000 units/mL, how many milliliters would Charlie prepare to give Mr. Santo?

2. What is the classification of the Bicillin-LA?

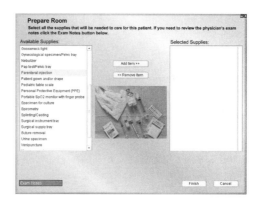
- In the Prepare Room wizard, click on **Parenteral Injection** found in the list of Available Supplies and review the contents on the tray shown in the photograph.

3. On the parenteral injection tray are four syringes, a tuberculin syringe, a 5-mL syringe, an insulin syringe, and a 3-mL syringe. Which is the correct syringe for the administration of the medication ordered?

4. Choose the correct syringe and mark to indicate the amount of medication that should be given to Mr. Santo.

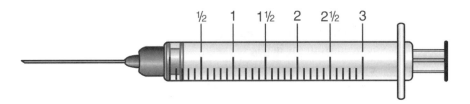

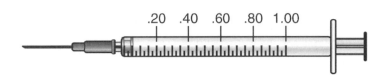

➡ • Click **Finish** to close the Prepare Room wizard and return to the Exam Room.

5. What is the correct disposal of the syringe following the administration of the Bicillin-LA?
   a. In a regular waste container
   b. In a biohazard waste container
   c. In a puncture-proof biohazard waste container

6. What is the proper disposal of the used supplies, other than the syringe, following the administration of Bicillin-LA?
   a. In a regular waste container
   b. In a biohazard waste container
   c. In a puncture-proof biohazard waste container

7. Properly document the injection given to Mr. Santo, using the date and time at present.

PATIENT'S NAME _____ ☐FEMALE ☐MALE Date of Birth: __/__/____	
DATE	PATIENT VISITS AND FINDINGS

ALLERGIC TO _____

PAGE _____ of _____

8. The Exam Notes state that the CBC should be drawn prior to the administration of the Bicillin-LA. Why should the CBC be drawn first and then the medication administered?

9. Why is it important for Mr. Santo to stay in the office for 15 to 20 minutes following the injection of Bicillin-LA?

10. The physician has stated in the Exam Notes that the patient should wait for 15 to 20 minutes before leaving the office. Mr. Santo was brought to the medical office by his employer, Mr. Freeman. If Mr. Freeman does not want to wait, what should the medical assistant at the check-out desk do?

 • Click the exit arrow to get to the Summary Menu.
- Select **Look at Your Performance Summary** to compare your answers for Jesus Santo with those of the experts.
- Select **Return to Map** to move on to the next exercise.

Exercise 2

 Online Activity—Administering and Documenting Immunizations

 30 minutes

- From the patient list, select **Shaunti Begay**. (*Note:* If you have exited the program, sign in again to Mountain View Clinic and select Shaunti Begay from the patient list.)

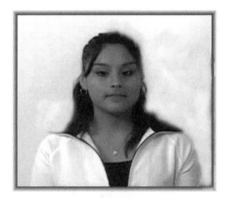

- On the office map, highlight and click on the **Exam Room**.

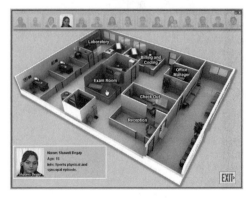

• Under the Watch heading, select **Immunizations** to view the video.

• At the end of the video, click **Close** to return to the Exam Room.

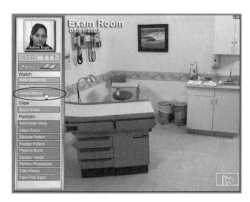

1. Where was the site of the hepatitis B immunization?

2. When is the next dose of hepatitis B due?

3. When the hepatitis B vaccine is being prepared for administration, when should the medical assistant check the medication against the physician's order prior to administering it?

 • Click the exit arrow to Return to Map.

• On the office map, highlight and click on **Check Out**.

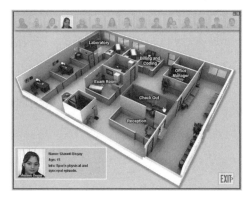

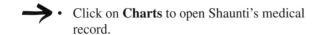

• Click on **Charts** to open Shaunti's medical record.

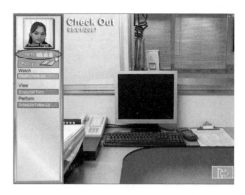

• Click on the **Patient Medical Information** tab and select **2-Progress Notes** to view the documentation of Shaunti's examination.
• Read the documentation regarding Shaunti's immunization.

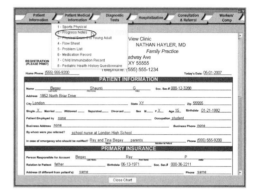

4. What volume of hepatitis B vaccine is being given to Shaunti?

5. Mark the diagram below to indicate the amount of vaccine that should be administered to Shaunti for the hepatitis B immunization.

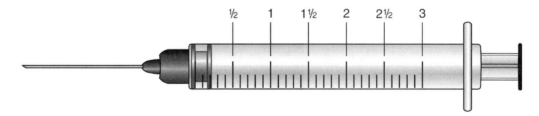

6. What is the expiration date of the hepatitis B vaccine?

7. What is a VIS statement? Why is this required for an immunization?

8. What are the seven rights of medication administration?

9. Why is it important to document the manufacturer of an immunizing agent, as well as the lot number and expiration date?

 • Click **Close Chart** to return to the Check Out area.
 • Click the exit arrow to get to the Summary Menu.
 • Click on **Return to Map** to continue to the next exercise.

Exercise 3

 Online Activity—Immunizations as Indicated in Well-Child Visits

 25 minutes

 • From the patient list, select **Jade Wong**. (*Note:* If you have exited the program, sign in again to Mountain View Clinic and select Jade Wong from the patient list.)

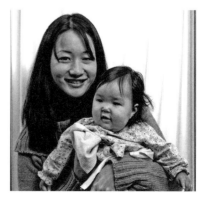

- On the office map, highlight and click on **Exam Room**.

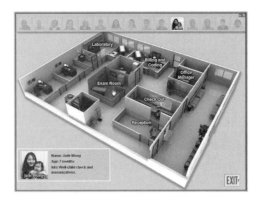

- Under the Watch heading, select **Immunizations** to view the video.

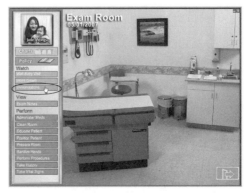

- At the end of the video, click **Close** to return to the Exam Room.
- Under the View heading, click on **Exam Notes** to read the documentation of Jade's visit.

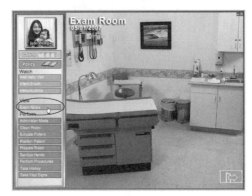

1. Why is it important to provide the parents with information, including the VIS, concerning the immunizations that the child will receive?

2. The medical assistant asked whether Jade had any problems with previous immunizations. Why is this information important before administering the immunizations at this visit?

3. What immunizations will be given to Jade? Be sure to include the diseases against which these immunizations protect (not just the abbreviations of the immunizations).

4. The Exam Notes indicate that Jade's mother has not received the polio vaccine. Why is the injectable polio vaccine safer for the mother?

5. What resources are available in your community for the mother to obtain the polio vaccine if she wants to get it some place other than the physician's office?

• Click on **Finish** to return to the Exam Room.

• Click on the exit arrow to get to the Summary Menu.

• On the Summary Menu, click on **Return to Map** to continue the lesson.

• On the office map, click on **Check Out** to review the end of Jade's visit.

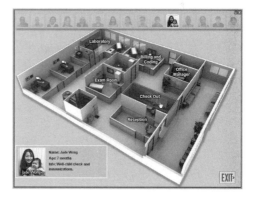

• At the Check Out desk, click on **Charts**. Next, click on the **Patient Medical Information** tab and select **1-Progress Notes**.

• Read the final documentation of Jade's examination.

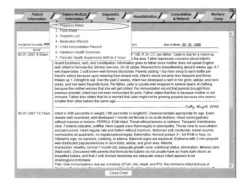

6. In the Progress Notes, the medical assistant states that Jade seemed to tolerate the immunizations with no problems. Why is this documentation important?

7. What volume of Pediarix will be administered to Jade?

8. Indicate on the syringe below the volume of Pediarix that Jade should receive.

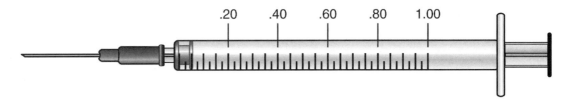

9. Below, document the immunizations that have been given to Jade today. Be sure to follow CDC guidelines.

Vaccine Administration Record for Children and Teens

Patient name: _____

Birthdate: _____

Chart number: _____

Before administering any vaccines, give the parent/guardian all appropriate copies of Vaccine Information Statements (VISs) and make sure they understand the risks and benefits of the vaccine(s). Update the patient's personal record card or provide a new one whenever you administer vaccine.

Vaccine	Type of Vaccine* (generic abbreviation)	Date given (mo/day/yr)	Route	Site given (RA, LA, RT, LT)	Vaccine		Vaccine Information Statement		Signature/ initials of vaccinator
					lot #	mfr.	Date on VIS§	Date given§	
Hepatitis B† (e.g., HepB, Hib-HepB, DTaP-HepB-IPV)			IM						
			IM						
			IM						
			IM						
Diphtheria, Tetanus, Pertussis† (e.g., DTaP, DT, DTaP-Hib, DTaP-HepB-IPV, Td)			IM						
			IM						
			IM						
			IM						
			IM						
			IM						
			IM						
Haemophilus influenzae type b† (e.g., Hib, Hib-HepB, DTaP-Hib)			IM						
			IM						
			IM						
			IM						
Polio† (e.g. IPV, DTaP-HepB-IPV)			IM•SC						
			IM•SC						
			IM•SC						
			IM•SC						
Pneumococcal conjugate (PCV)			IM						
			IM						
			IM						
			IM						
Measles, Mumps, Rubella (MMR)			SC						
			SC						
Varicella (Var)			SC						
			SC						
Hepatitis A** (HepA)			IM						
			IM						
Influenza** (Flu)			IM						
			IM						
			IM						
			IM						
			IM						
Other**									
Other**									

*Record the generic abbreviation for the type of vaccine given (e.g., DTaP-Hib, PCV), *not* the trade name.

†For combination vaccines, fill in the row for each individual antigen composing the combination.

§Record the publication date of each VIS as well as the date it is given to the patient. According to federal law, VISs must be given to patients (or parent/guardian of a minor child) before administering each dose of DTaP, Td, Hib, polio, MMR, varicella, PCV, or HepB vaccine, or combinations thereof.

**Influenza, pneumococcal polysaccharide (PPV23), hepatitis A, and/or meningococcal vaccines are recommended for certain high-risk children.

www.immunize.org/catg.d/p2022b.pdf • Item #P2022 (4/03)

Immunization Action Coalition • 1573 Selby Avenue • St. Paul, MN 55104 • (651) 647-9009 • www.immunize.org

10. Why is the use of a 1-mL syringe more appropriate when administering the medication to Jade?

- Click **Close Chart** to return to the Check Out desk.
- Under the **Watch** heading, select **Patient Check-Out** to view the video.

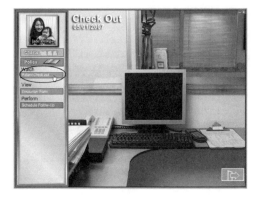

11. The medical assistant provides Jade's father, Mr. Wong, with information concerning child nutrition and community resources. She indicates that Mr. Wong and his wife are open to this help. Why is it important that the implied permission is provided, either verbally or nonverbally, prior to giving information?

12. The Progress Notes also state that Jade's mother has been referred to ESL classes. What does ESL mean?

13. Using the Internet or a resource guide, list the resources for ESL education in your area.

Fecal Specimen Collection

📖 **Reading Assignment:** Chapter 39—Assisting in Gastroenterology
- The Medical Assistant's Role in the Gastrointestinal Examination

Patient: John R. Simmons

Learning Objectives:

- Understand the reasons for collecting fecal specimens.
- Using the package insert of the fecal occult test, identify the correct steps to give the patient when providing patient education for preparing and collecting the specimen.
- Describe the development of the fecal occult test and the visual appearance of the controls.
- Identify the possible indications of a positive fecal occult test.
- Understand the need for quality control when obtaining and testing a fecal specimen.

Overview:

In this lesson Dr. John R. Simmons, a college professor, will be asked to provide the medical office with fecal specimens to be tested for occult blood. The medical assistant has the responsibility of providing Dr. Simmons with the necessary preparation to ensure that a quality test will be obtained. Dr. Simmons has not been asked to do this test previously, so specific instructions must be provided. Discussing fecal specimens tends to embarrass most patients, so it is important that the medical assistant respond with dignity and professionalism. Furthermore, it is imperative that the correct instructions be given; otherwise, the patient may provide a specimen that cannot be tested.

Exercise 1

Online Activity—Patient Instruction for Collecting Fecal Specimens

40 minutes

- Sign in to Mountain View Clinic.
- Select **John R. Simmons** from the patient list.

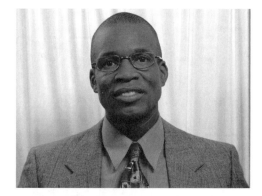

- On the office map, highlight and click on **Exam Room** to enter the examination area.

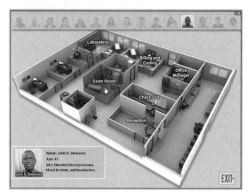

- Under the **Watch** heading, select **Patient Instruction** to observe the video.

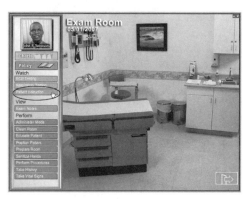

1. Dr. Simmons seems embarrassed by the need to collect stool specimens. How did the medical assistant attempt to put him at ease?

2. What is a guaiac test? How is this test related to fecal specimens?

3. Which of the following supplies do patients need to obtain fecal specimens at home? Select all that apply.

_____   Gloves

_____   Wooden applicator sticks

_____   Test kits (the number is based on the physician's policy)

_____   Plastic wrap

_____   Written instructions

_____   Addressed envelope

Go to your Evolve account and enter the course area for this textbook. Under the Course Documents heading, access the document "Fecal Occult Testing Kit Package Insert." This is one type of fecal occult testing kit. Answer the following questions using the package insert.

4. Which of the following should the medical assistant tell the patient when providing instructions for preparing to obtain a fecal specimen? Select all that apply.

_____ Avoid all vegetables for 3 days.

_____ Eat a high-fiber diet for 3 days.

_____ Do not eat red meat, including processed meats and cold cuts, for 3 days.

_____ Take all medications ordered by the physician.

_____ Avoid taking aspirin, corticosteroids, and NSAIDs for a week before collecting the specimen.

_____ Do not collect stool specimens during a menstrual period or for 3 days afterward.

_____ Eat foods that will cause softening of stools to make the specimen easier to obtain.

_____ Eat small amounts of food that contain vitamin C.

_____ Do not eat raw fruits and vegetables, especially melons, radishes, turnips, and horseradish.

_____ Eat cooked vegetables.

_____ Drink at least three glasses of milk per day.

_____ Do not take iron or vitamin C for 3 days.

_____ Eat moderate amounts of bran cereal, popcorn, and other roughage.

5. When test kits are taken home, how should the patient store the kits until the specimens are collected?

6. What directions should be given to the patient about the timing of specimens?

7. Which of the following are correct instructions to give to the patient about obtaining the stool specimen? Select all that apply.

_____ Using the wooden applicator stick, collect a sample of stool either from a container or from toilet paper.

_____ If the stool falls in the commode, collect the sample as you would from the container or the toilet paper.

_____ Open the flap of the first kit on the left (be sure there are two square boxes inside, labeled A and B); then smear a small amount of stool on the filter paper labeled A, making sure to spread it until thin.

_____ Using the same wooden stick, collect a second sample of stool from another area of the stool.

_____ Place this sample on top of the sample already collected.

_____ Place the second sample in the filter paper box labeled B.

_____ Close the front flap.

_____ Tear this test kit from the other two and place it in the envelope provided.

_____ Add the date and time of collection on the flap.

_____ Repeat the same procedure with the next two stools (if three test kits were provided).

_____ Allow the specimens to air-dry before mailing to the office.

_____ Place the specimens in a standard letter-sized envelope and mail.

_____ Place the specimens in an aluminum-lined envelope designed for sending to the medical office.

8. Why is it important that the smears be taken from two different areas of the stool?

9. Why is it important that the patient add roughage to the diet?

10. On the form below, document the procedure for instructing the patient in the collection of a fecal specimen.

PATIENT'S NAME	☐ FEMALE ☐ MALE Date of Birth: ___/___/___
DATE	**PATIENT VISITS AND FINDINGS**

ALLERGIC TO _____

_____ PAGE _____ of _____

Exercise 2

Writing Activity—Developing a Hemoccult Slide Test

20 minutes

A week after his visit, Dr. John R. Simmons has returned the Hemoccult slides to the medical office for development. In this exercise, you will describe the steps necessary to develop the test and provide documentation to the physician.

1. Which of the following are the proper supplies needed for developing the Hemoccult test? Select all that apply.

_____ Sterile gloves

_____ Gloves

_____ Gown and goggles

_____ Developer solution

_____ Wooden sticks

_____ Watch

_____ Reference card

_____ Biohazard waste container

2. Now that you have chosen the proper supplies for developing the Hemoccult, match the following columns to show the correct order of the steps.

Order		Action
_____	Step 1	a. Ensure quality control by checking the expiration date on slides and developer.
_____	Step 2	
		b. Don the correct personal protective equipment.
_____	Step 3	
		c. Dispose of the used Hemoccult slides in a proper waste container.
_____	Step 4	
_____	Step 5	d. Read the results in 60 seconds.
_____	Step 6	e. Open the back flap of the slides.
_____	Step 7	f. Document the results in the medical record.
_____	Step 8	g. Sanitize hands following the procedure.
_____	Step 9	h. Sanitize hands before the procedure.
_____	Step 10	i. Compare the results with the reference card.
		j. Apply two drops of developing solution to the guaiac test paper and the quality control area.

3. Why is it important to read the Hemoccult slide results at the end of 60 seconds?

4. The result of the first specimen obtained by Dr. Simmons was negative, but slides 2 and 3 were positive. Document these results on the Progress Notes below.

PATIENT'S NAME	☐FEMALE ☐MALE Date of Birth: ___/___/___
DATE	PATIENT VISITS AND FINDINGS

ALLERGIC TO _____

PAGE _____ of _____

5. What does a positive Hemoccult test indicate?

6. What are the indications if the positive quality control area does not change to a blue color?

7. What are two possible causes of invalid tests?

Assisting with a Prenatal/ Gynecological Examination

Reading Assignment: Chapter 41—Assisting in Obstetrics and Gynecology
- Pregnancy
- The Medical Assistant's Role in Gynecological and Obstetric Procedures

Patients: Renee Anderson, Louise Parlet

Learning Objectives:

- Choose the necessary questions to ask the patient to obtain information for a thorough health history and gynecological and prenatal examinations.
- Understand the appropriate positions in which the patient will be placed for the gynecological examination
- Discuss the legal and ethical boundaries of preparing a patient for a gynecological/prenatal examination.
- Discuss the legal and ethical issues associated with assault/domestic abuse.
- Document the patient information into the medical record.
- Understand how a medical assistant should handle domestic abuse concerns ethically and professionally.
- Assess how verbal and nonverbal communications are important to assess with victims of domestic abuse.
- Read a health history form to obtain information that may indicate the patient has been abused.

Overview:

This lesson is designed around two patients, Louise Parlet, an established patient who is having a routine prenatal examination, and Renee Anderson, a new patient coming in for a routine gynecological examination. Ms. Anderson is also a victim of domestic abuse.

Exercise 1

Online Activity—Assisting with a Routine Prenatal Examination

45-60 minutes

- Sign in to Mountain View Clinic.
- From the patient list, select **Louise Parlet**.

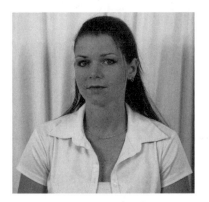

- On the office map, highlight and click on **Exam Room**.

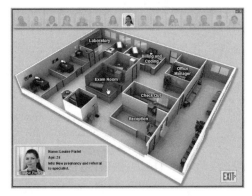

- In the Exam Room, click on **Exam Notes** to view the documentation for this visit.

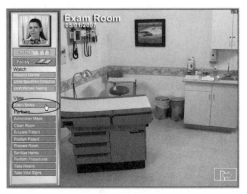

- Click on **Finish** to close the Exam Notes and return to the Exam Room.
- Under the Perform heading, click on **Prepare Room** to select the supplies needed for Louise Parlet's visit. (*Note:* You can reopen the Exam Notes for reference as you make your selections.)

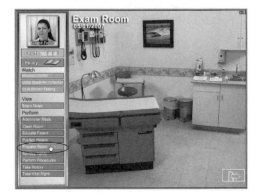

- Select the first item needed for Ms. Parlet's visit from the alphabetical list and click **Add Item** to confirm your choice. The items you select will appear in the Selected Supplies column.

- Repeat this step until you are satisfied you have everything you need from the list.

- Do not close this window. Keep the Prepare Room wizard open as you continue with the lesson.

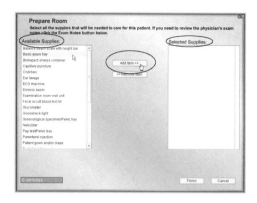

1. Match the columns below to indicate the order in which you will use the items needed for a gynecological examination.

Order of Use	**Item**
_____ First	a. Water-soluble lubricant
_____ Second	b. Cytobrush/spatula
_____ Third	c. Laboratory requisition form
_____ Fourth	d. Gloves for the physician
_____ Fifth	e. Speculum
_____ Sixth	f. Gloves for the medical assistant
_____ Seventh	g. Culture transport, if applicable

- Returning to the open Prepare Room wizard, confirm that you have chosen the necessary supplies for Ms. Parlet's Pap smear. When you click on an item, a photograph of that item will appear, which can be used for reference as you review your list of supplies.

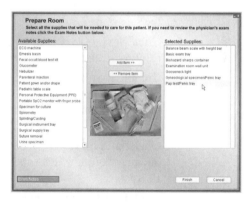

- After completing all the selections you wish to make, click **Finish** to return to the Exam Room.

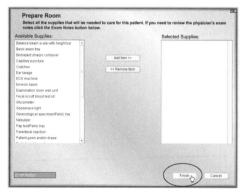

• Remain in the Exam Room with Louise Parlet. Under the Perform heading, click on **Position Patient**.

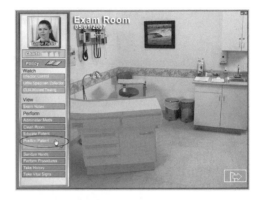

• Select all positions in which Ms. Parlet will be placed during her examination.
• Click **Finish** to return to the Exam Room.

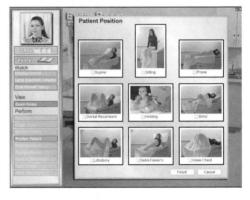

2. Practice documenting in the patient's medical record by following these steps.

• While still in the Exam Room, click on **Take History**.
• Click on the **Ask** button to view Ms. Parlet's answers to the questions regarding her medical history. Document your findings as directed in the program.
• Click **Next** to view additional questions and responses related to her history.
• Complete your documentation in the program. (*Note:* You can return to the previous page to review Ms. Parlet's answers without losing your work.)
• Click on **Print** to get a hard copy of your documentation, which can be turned in to your instructor.
• Click **Finish** to return to the Exam Room.

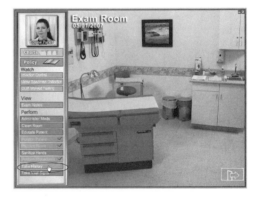

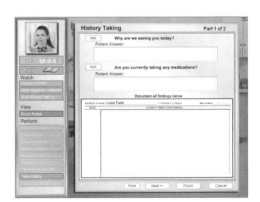

3. What information is important to obtain before a prenatal examination?

4. What information did Ms. Parlet provide that might indicate that she is pregnant?

5. How many times has Ms. Parlet conceived? What was the outcome?

Thought Questions

6. Why might a patient who has previously had a spontaneous abortion be "afraid" of complications of pregnancy and therefore phone the office more frequently with questions than other patients who are pregnant?

7. What are ways the medical assistant can alleviate apprehension and provide emotional support to these patients?

8. List the positions used for Ms. Parlet's examination in the order they will be used.

   (1)

   (2)

   (3)

9. Explain the use of each of the positions chosen.

➤ • Remain in the Exam Room with Louise Parlet.
  • Click on **Perform Procedures** and open the Exam Notes to review which procedures are to be performed on Ms. Parlet for this visit.

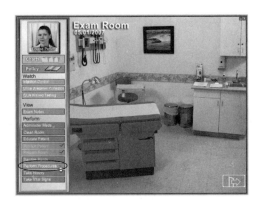

• Select all procedures that should be performed on Ms. Parlet during her visit.
 • Click **Finish** to return to the Exam Room.

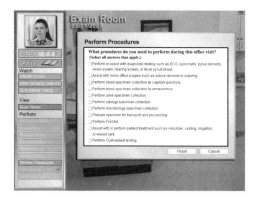

10. Which procedures were accomplished? Why were these needed for the prenatal examination?

 • Click the exit arrow to get to the Summary Menu.
 • Click on **Look at Your Performance Summary**.
 • Scroll through the sections to view each area you completed and compare your answers with those of the experts. The summary can also be printed or saved for your instructor. Click on **Close** to return to the Summary Menu.
 • Click on **Return to Map** to begin the next exercise.

Exercise 2

 Online Activity—Assisting with a Gynecological Examination

 30 minutes

 • From the patient list, select **Renee Anderson**. (*Note:* If you have exited the program, sign in again to Mountain View Clinic and select Renee Anderson from the patient list.)

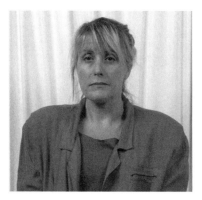

→ • On the office map, highlight **Reception** and click to enter the Reception area.

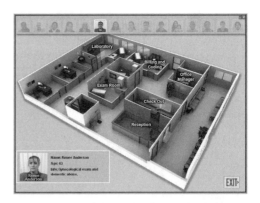

• Click on **Patient Check-In** to watch the video.
• Click **Close** to return to the Reception desk.

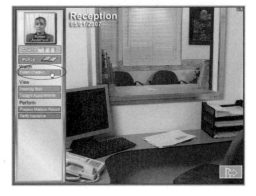

1. What nonverbal communication is most important in this video for the medical assistant to observe and respond to?

2. Did the medical assistant at check-in handle the confidentiality question correctly and accurately? Explain your answer.

• At the Reception desk, click on **Prepare Medical Record** to assemble a chart for Ms. Anderson.

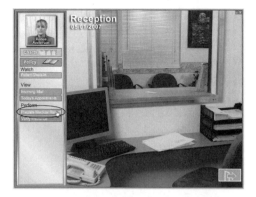

• Select **Perform: Assemble Medical Record** to select the forms necessary for Ms. Anderson's visit. The Patient Information tab will appear on top.

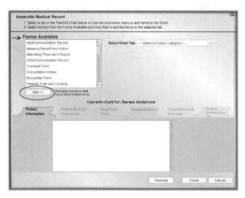

• From the list of Forms Available, highlight each form that should be filed under the Patient Information tab. Click on **Add** to confirm your choices.

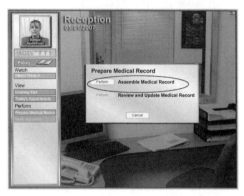

• When this tab is complete, continue adding forms to the appropriate tabs in Ms. Anderson's medical record. To select a new tab, either click on the tab on the medical record itself or use the drop-down menu next to Select Chart Tab.

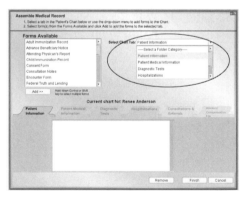

- If you change your mind about a form you have added to a tab, click to highlight the name of the form and then click **Remove** at the bottom of the screen.

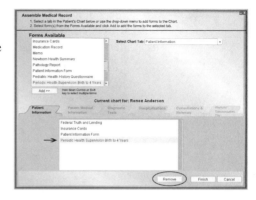

- After selecting and filing all the necessary forms under the correct tabs, click **Finish** to close the medical record.

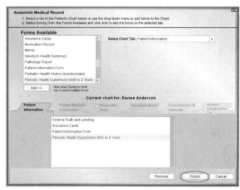

- Exit from the reception area.
- Click **Return to Map** to continue with this exercise.

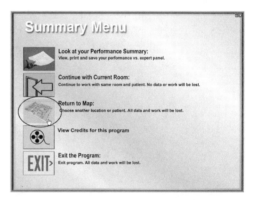

- With Renee Anderson as the patient, click on **Exam Room** on the office map.

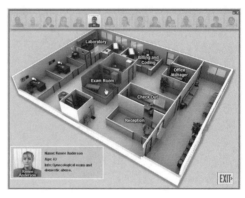

- Under the Watch heading, click on **Patient Care** to view the video.
- At the end of the video, click **Close** to return to the Exam Room.

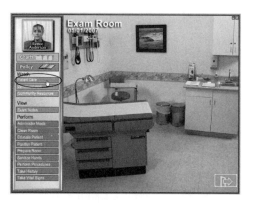

3. In the video, Susan states that she missed a question on the laboratory request form concerning previously abnormal Pap smears. Why is this important?

4. During the examination, what nonverbal communication did the patient provide to the medical assistant and physician that might have led to an examination for spousal abuse by the physician?

5. Do you think Susan provided the appropriate verbal and nonverbal support for a patient whose nonverbal communication at check-in indicated an emotional problem? Explain.

6. Why is it important to include the instructions for breast self-examination with each gynecological patient?

→ • From the Exam Room, click on **Charts**.

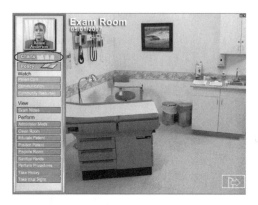

• Under the **Patient Medical Information** tab, choose **General Health History Questionnaire** from the drop-down menu and read the document in its entirety. (*Note:* To move from page to page, click on the oval at the top right side of each page.)

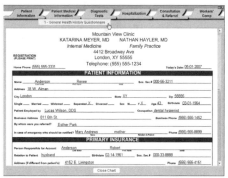

7. Dr. Hayler suggests that Ms. Anderson have a mammogram. Other than finding a breast lump, what reason would be appropriate for suggesting this mammogram? (*Hint:* Check the Patient Information Form in her chart for age and health history.)

8. Along with the physical findings documented on page 6 of the health history form, what additional information on the form provides a hint of spousal abuse?

- Click on **Close Chart** to return to the Exam Room.
- Click on **Communication** under the Watch heading to view the video.
- At the end of the video, click **Close** to return to the Exam Room.

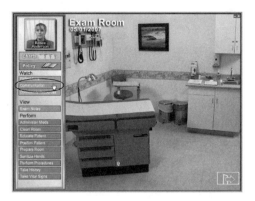

9. When Ms. Anderson arrived for her appointment, ethical and confidential matters were discussed. What did Dr. Hayler and the medical assistant do to continue the ethical and confidential manner of the examination?

10. How do you feel about the manner that Dr. Hayler used when talking with Ms. Anderson, as well as the response of the medical assistant, Susan, to the patient's nonverbal communication?

11. What responsibilities did the medical assistant have concerning the cleaning of the room before Dr. Hayler returned to discuss treatment with Ms. Anderson?

- From the Exam Room, choose **Clean Room**. Select the things that Susan will need to do to clean the room.
- Click **Finish** when you have chosen the required tasks.

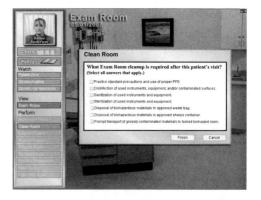

- Click on the exit arrow at the bottom of screen to leave the Reception area. On the Summary Menu, click on **Look at Your Performance Summary** to compare your answers with those of the experts.
- Click **Close** to return to the Summary Menu.

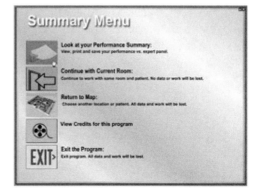

Critical Thinking Question

12. What should be the next step in caring for a patient who may be the victim of domestic abuse?

13. Indicate whether each of the following statements is true or false.

a. _____ The date of the last menstrual period is not important on the laboratory requisition form for a Pap smear.

b. _____ The medical assistant is responsible for asking the site of specimen collection during a Pap smear if this information is not provided by the physician.

c. _____ When assisting with a pelvic examination, the medical assistant should be near the supply tray to pass needed supplies to the physician but should also be at the side of the patient to provide support and to observe nonverbal communication.

d. _____ With a female patient and a male examiner, the medical assistant has a legal and ethical responsibility to remain in the room at all times.

Assisting with a Pediatric Examination

Reading Assignment: Chapter 5—Interpersonal Skills and Human Behavior
- Multicultural Issues

Chapter 42—Assisting in Pediatrics
- Normal Growth and Development
- Immunizations
- The Pediatric Patient
- The Medical Assistant's Role in Pediatric Procedures

Patient: Jade Wong

Learning Objectives:

- Describe the steps necessary in preparing a child for a pediatric examination.
- Identify similarities and differences when obtaining mensurations in children and in adults.
- Plot height and weight on a growth chart for children, and identify trends in percentile ranking.
- Describe the role of the medical assistant in a pediatric examination.
- Understand the importance of effective verbal and nonverbal communication with persons of different cultures.
- Understand methods of parental involvement while preparing infants for a physical examination.
- Read the Progress Notes to obtain information about the patient's visit.

Overview:

In this lesson students will be introduced to the pediatric examination and will be expected to identify the differences in examining a pediatric patient versus an adult patient. Jade Wong's parents are of Asian descent and speak little English. During Jade's pediatric visit, the medical assistant explains the needs to the father, who acts as an interpreter. The mother is also provided with information concerning immunizations for health promotion and disease prevention.

Exercise 1

Online Activity—Assisting with a Pediatric Examination

 45 minutes

- Sign in to Mountain View Clinic.
- From the patient list, select **Jade Wong**.

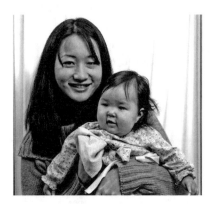

- On the office map, highlight and click on **Reception** to enter the Reception area.

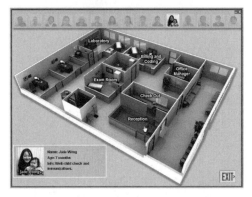

- Under the Perform heading, click on **Prepare Medical Record**.

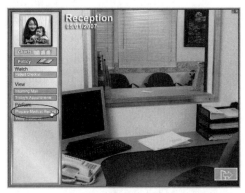

- Select **Perform: Assemble Medical Record** to select the forms necessary for Jade's visit. The Patient Information Tab will open automatically.

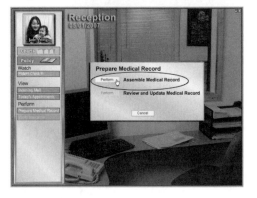

- From the Forms Available list, choose the forms that should be filed under the Patient Information tab. Click on **Add** to confirm your choice.

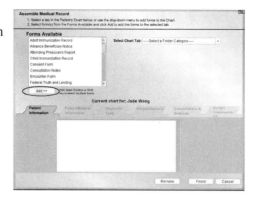

- When the Patient Information tab is complete, move to each of the other tabs that you think are necessary to prepare this patient's medical record. To select a new tab, you may either click on the tab on the medical record or use the drop-down menu next to Select Chart Tab. Continue selecting forms to fill the tabs in Jade Wong's medical record.

- If you wish to remove a chosen form, highlight the form and click the **Remove** button.

- After selecting and filing all the necessary forms under the correct tabs, click **Finish** to close the chart.

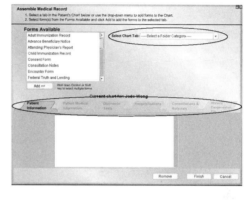

- Click on the exit arrow at the bottom of screen to leave the Reception area. From the Summary Menu, select **Look at Your Performance Summary** to compare your answers with those of the experts. How did you do?

- Click **Close** to return to the Summary Menu.

- Click **Return to Map** to continue with this exercise.

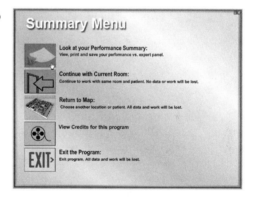

- Keeping Jade Wong as the patient, click on **Exam Room** on the office map.

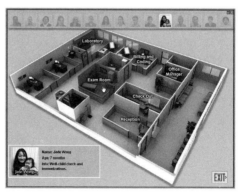

• Under the Watch heading, select **Well-Baby Visit** and watch the video.
 • Click **Close** at the end of the video to return to the Exam Room.

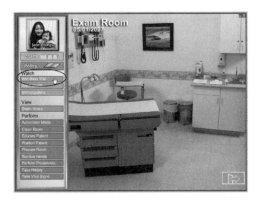

1. What measurements would you expect the medical assistant to obtain on Jade for a well-baby visit? How does this differ from an adult measurement?

2. Why is it important for the medical assistant to develop rapport with a child and with parents when assisting with a well-child office visit?

3. As the medical assistant works with Jade, she is using the father as an interpreter and is allowing the mother to have an active part in the medical care through this means. Do you feel this is an important part of the care, or do you believe the medical assistant should provide care and speak only with the father? Explain your answer.

4. Why is it important to remove the clothing on the infant prior to weight taking? Why should the diaper be removed?

Critical Thinking Question

5. What are some of the differences between the preparation of a 4-year-old child for an examination versus the preparation of an adult for an examination?

6. What tactics may be used with older children to gain their confidence?

7. What roles do verbal communication and nonverbal communication play in a pediatric examination?

→ • Remain in the Exam Room with Jade and select **Position Patient** under the Perform heading.

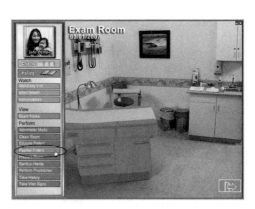

- Select all positions Jade will be placed in during her exam.
- When you have made all your selections, click **Finish**.

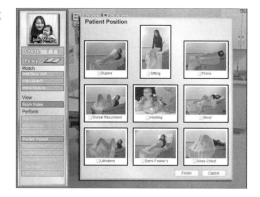

- Under the Watch heading, click on **Infant Growth** and watch the video.
- Click **Close** to return to the Exam Room.
- Click the exit arrow to go to the Summary Menu.
- On the Summary Menu, click on **Look at Your Performance Summary**.
- Scroll down to the relevant section and compare your patient position selections with those of the experts. The summary can be printed or saved for your instructor.
- Click **Close** to return to the Summary Menu.
- Click on **Return to Map** to continue the lesson.
- Continue with Jade Wong as the patient. On the office map, highlight and click on **Billing and Coding**. (*Note:* You will need to be in the Billing and Coding area to view the Progress Notes. They cannot be accessed from the Exam Room.)

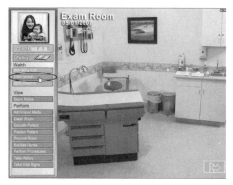

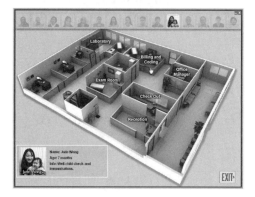

- Open Jade's records by clicking on **Charts**.

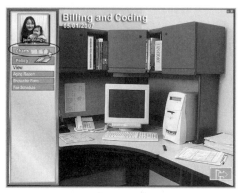

- Click on the **Patient Medical Information** tab and select **2-Newborn Health Summary** to review some of Jade's past medical history.

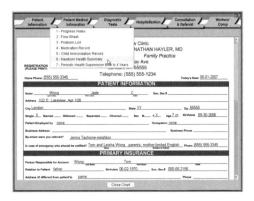

8. Record Jade's birth weight and length from the medical history in the Newborn Health Summary.

- Click again on the **Patient Medical Information** tab and select **1-Progress Notes**.

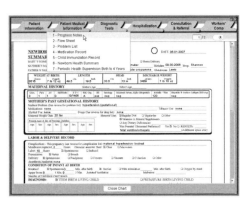

9. What measurements were recorded from today's visit?

- Look again at the Progress Notes in the Billing and Coding area of the office and read the chief complaint documented for today's visit.

10. Why is the chief complaint in quotation marks?

11. Indicate whether each of the following statements is true or false.

a. _____ The growth charts are the same for both genders and for all ages.

b. _____ A well-baby visit is usually scheduled every 2 months for the first 6 months so that the child can receive the needed immunizations on schedule.

c. _____ After the age of 6 months, well-baby visits are scheduled every 3 months until age 18 months.

d. _____ After 2 years of age, well-child visits are scheduled every 2 years.

e. _____ The medical assistant should obtain information about the motor and cognitive development of the child at each visit.

f. _____ If a child is seen for a sick-child visit between well-baby visits, the child does not need to have weight and length obtained.

g. _____ When measuring the circumference of the head and chest, each measurement should be taken at the site of greatest circumference.

h. _____ Infant scales measure weight in pounds and ounces rather than in pounds and fractions of pounds as with adult scales.

i. _____ When measuring the height of an infant, the measurement should be from the heel to the crown of the head.

j. _____ When a child is able to stand, the child may be weighed on balance beam scales with no difficulty.

k. _____ When weighing a young child who is afraid of the balance beam scales or who weighs more than the infant scale can accommodate, an alternative is to weigh the mother and child together on an adult scale and then weigh the mother alone. After obtaining the two weights, you can determine the weight of the child by subtracting the mother's weight from the combined weight of the two.

Exercise 2

Writing Activity—Plotting a Growth Chart and Recognizing Trends in Percentiles

20 minutes

1. On the next page, plot the growth chart for Kaitlynn Griffin using these measurements.

3 months	22¾ inches	11 pounds
6 months	26 inches	14 pounds, 8 ounces
9 months	27½ inches	16 pounds, 4 ounces
13 months	30½ inches	19 pounds
16 months	31½ inches	20 pounds, 8 ounces
24 months	34¾ inches	27 pounds

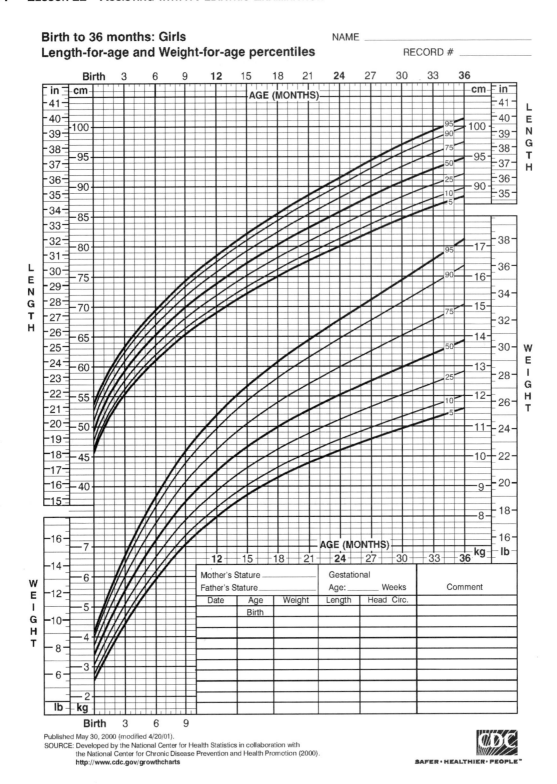

Birth to 36 months: Girls
Length-for-age and Weight-for-age percentiles

NAME _____

RECORD # _____

Published May 30, 2000 (modified 4/20/01).
SOURCE: Developed by the National Center for Health Statistics in collaboration with
the National Center for Chronic Disease Prevention and Health Promotion (2000).
http://www.cdc.gov/growthcharts

2. Compare Kaitlynn's percentiles. What trend do you see on her length?

3. What trend did you see in her weight gain?

23

Respiratory Testing

✎ **Reading Assignment:** Chapter 46—Assisting in Pulmonary Medicine
  • The Medical Assistant's Role in Pulmonary Procedures

Patients: John R. Simmons, Hu Huang

Learning Objectives:

• Understand the purpose of pulmonary function tests.
• Be familiar with abbreviations associated with pulmonary function tests and their definitions.
• Identify pulmonary function tests performed in the physician's office.
• Identify contraindications for spirometry testing.
• Distinguish between lung function tests.
• Identify the necessary steps in patient preparation for respiratory testing.
• Understand the unique role of the medical assistant in spirometry testing.
• Identify possible reasons for obtaining a sputum specimen.
• Correctly document the spirometry results into the patient's Progress Notes of the health record.

Overview:

This lesson is designed to provide instruction in respiratory testing and the proper documentation of the procedure. Dr. John R. Simmons, a college professor, will have respiratory testing as a part of his complete medical examination. Another patient, Hu Huang, has a suspected diagnosis of avian flu that he may have acquired during a trip to Asia. He will be providing sputum specimens for a differential diagnosis. Standard precautions will be necessary while performing the test and when discarding supplies following the testing and sputum collection.

Exercise 1

Writing Activity—Elements in Respiratory Testing

15 minutes

1. What are the purposes of pulmonary function tests?

2. Identify the method of testing pulmonary function in the physician's office setting?

3. List at least three indications for spirometry testing.

4. Match each spirometry testing term with its correct definition.

Term	**Definition**
_____ Maximum volume ventilation (MVV)	a. Amount of air that can be forcefully exhaled from a maximum inhalation
_____ Functional residual volume (FRV)	b. Volume of air left in the lungs after a forced expiration
_____ Expiratory reserve volume (ERV)	c. Maximum amount of air that can be expired after a maximum inspiration
_____ Residual volume (RV)	d. Maximum volume the patient can breathe in and out in 1 minute
_____ Forced vital capacity (FVC)	
_____ Vital capacity (VC)	e. Volume of air inspired and expired during a normal respiration
_____ Inspiratory capacity (IC)	f. Maximum amount of air that can be expired after a normal inspiration
_____ Tidal volume (TV)	g. Amount of air left in the lungs after a normal expiration
	h. Maximum volume of air that can be exhaled after a normal inspiration

Exercise 2

Online Activity—Preparing the Patient and Performing Spirometry Testing

30 minutes

- Sign in to Mountain View Clinic.
- From the patient list, select **John R. Simmons**.

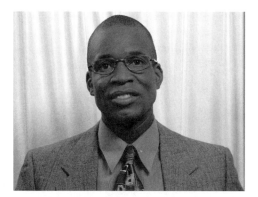

- Highlight and click on **Exam Room** to enter the examination area.

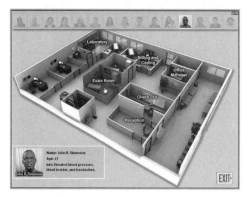

- Under the Watch heading, click on **Respiratory Testing** to view the video.

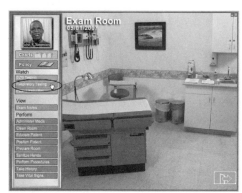

1. What preparation of the patient was provided during the video?

2. During the video, Dr. Simmons asks the medical assistant what the "contraption" is. What would be the proper answer to his question?

3. What other instructions should be given to patients who are preparing to come to the medical office for spirometry testing?

4. What is the proper position for spirometry testing, and why is this important?

5. How many attempts should the patient be given to obtain quality testing?

6. During the testing, what should the medical assistant do to encourage an acceptable test?

- Click **Close** at the end of the video to return to the Exam Room.
- Click on **Exam Notes** to view the documentation of Dr. Simmons' current visit.

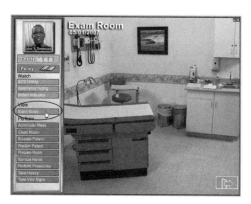

7. What vital signs should the medical assistant record prior to spirometry testing?

8. Indicate whether each of the following statements is true or false.

a. _____ During the video, the medical assistant provided the needed information for Dr. Simmons to obtain an acceptable test.

b. _____ The patient's lips may be loosely pursed around the mouthpiece without affecting the results of the test.

c. _____ The medical assistant should obtain the patient's height and weight before performing the test for computerized spirometers to make the correct calculations.

d. _____ When the test is completed, the mouthpiece may be reused.

e. _____ The medical assistant should provide coaching only while the patient is exhaling air into the mouthpiece.

9. On the blank Progress Notes below, document Dr. Simmons' spirometry testing, including his results of 85%, 90%, and 78% on the peak flow testing.

PATIENT'S NAME	☐FEMALE ☐MALE Date of Birth: / /
DATE	PATIENT VISITS AND FINDINGS

ALLERGIC TO _____

PAGE _____ of _____

10. Continue reviewing the written documentation of Dr. Simmons' testing in the Exam Notes. Which documentation would be more helpful to the physician—the notes with the readings of the spirometry testing or the Exam Notes?

➡ • Click **Finish** to return to the Exam Room.
 • Click the exit arrow to go to the Summary Menu.
 • Click **Return to Map** and continue to Exercise 3.

Exercise 3

Online Activity—Collecting Sputum Specimens

 15 minutes

• Select **Hu Huang** from the patient list.

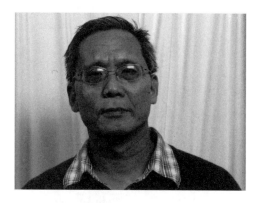

• On the office map, highlight and click on **Exam Room**.

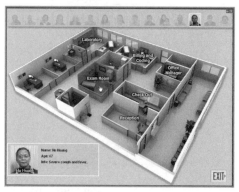

• Under Watch, click on **Sputum Collection** to view the video.

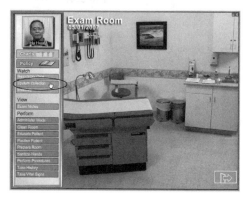

1. What directions should be provided to the patient before obtaining a sputum specimen?

2. Why are sputum specimens usually collected?

3. What types of testing are usually performed on sputum tests?

4. Which of the following PPE and other supplies are essential for preventing cross-contamination when obtaining a sputum specimen? Select all that apply.

_____ Sterile gloves

_____ Gloves

_____ Gown

_____ Goggles/face shield

_____ Shoe covers

_____ Mask

_____ Table covering

_____ Puncture-proof biohazard container

_____ Biohazard waste bag

5. On the blank form below, document the collection of Hu Huang's sputum specimen using today's date, time, and your name.

PATIENT'S NAME		☐ FEMALE ☐ MALE Date of Birth: ___/___/___
DATE	**PATIENT VISITS AND FINDINGS**	

ALLERGIC TO _____

_____ PAGE _____ of _____

Electrocardiogram

Reading Assignment: Chapter 47—Assisting in Cardiology
- Anatomy of the Heart
- Diagnostic Procedures and Treatments
- Diseases and Disorders of the Heart

Chapter 49—Principles of Electrocardiography
- The Electrical Conduction System of the Heart
- The Electrocardiograph
- Performing Electrocardiography
- Interpreting an ECG Strip

Patient: John R. Simmons

Learning Objectives:

- Discuss the purpose of electrocardiography (ECG).
- Explain when Holter monitoring would be indicated.
- Identify the correct placement of leads for an ECG.
- Identify the waves, segments, and intervals that show up on an ECG that are representative of the cardiac cycle.
- State the need for quality control and the use of standardization marks when performing ECGs.
- Discuss the proper way to handle ECG paper.
- Describe patient preparation for an ECG.
- Identify the 12 leads found on an electrocardiogram.
- Understand what an artifact is and what causes it.
- Discuss ways of maintaining professionalism and ethical behavior to make a patient more comfortable when performing electrocardiography.
- Identify what modifications in lead placement should be made if the patient has amputations, wounds, or injuries.
- Document correctly that an ECG was performed on a patient.

Overview:

In this lesson Dr. John R. Simmons, a college professor, will have a routine electrocardiogram. You will be asked to show your knowledge of the heart and to discuss the means of testing the electrical activity of the heart.

Exercise 1

Writing Activity—Basic Anatomy of the Heart and Risk Factors

15 minutes

1. The heart has _____ chambers. The top chambers are called _____,

   and the bottom chambers are called _____.

2. The heart is about the same size as an adult's _____.

3. The average adult heart pumps about _____ liters of blood every minute.

4. The sac that encloses the heart is called the _____.

5. _____ located between the chambers of the heart help ensure that blood
   flows from one chamber to another as it should.

6. List four risk factors for heart disease that cannot be changed.

   (1)

   (2)

   (3)

   (4)

7. List six risk factors for heart disease that can be modified or treated.

   (1)

   (2)

   (3)

   (4)

   (5)

   (6)

Exercise 2

**Writing Activity—Understanding the Purpose and Components of an
Electrocardiogram**

45 minutes

1. What is electrocardiography?

2. What does the electrocardiograph machine measure?

3. Define "cardiac cycle."

4. In an adult, what is the average length of the cardiac cycle?

5. Label the diagram below to show the main structures of the heart.

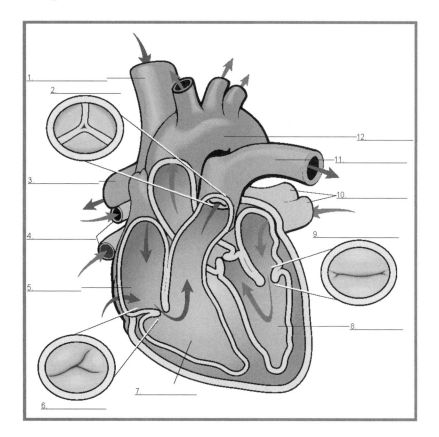

6. Label the waves, segments, and intervals on the ECG tracing below.

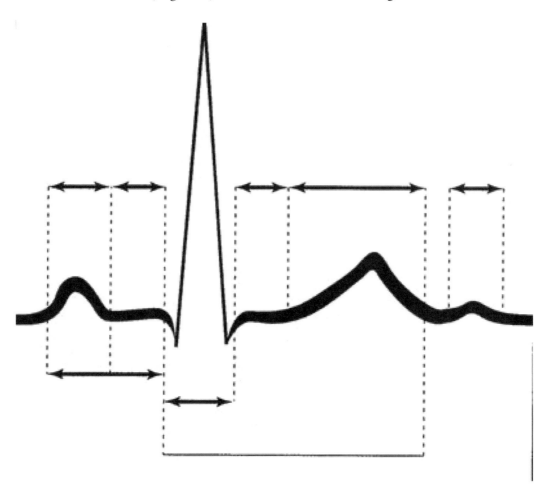

7. What does a wave in an electrocardiogram tracing indicate?

8. What does the ST segment in an electrocardiogram tracing indicate?

9. What does the QT interval on an electrocardiogram tracing indicate?

10. What does the QRS complex indicate on an electrocardiogram tracing?

11. How does the physician use electrocardiograph paper to interpret the tracing?

12. Why is it important that the ECG tracing be handled carefully and not be allowed to smear or be folded in any way?

13. What is the purpose of the standardization mark on an electrocardiogram? How is it used?

14. a. When the electrical impulse arrives and the heart muscle is ready to contract, this is called _____.

b. When the electrical impulse is received and the heart muscle contracts, this is called

_____.

c. When the electrical impulse ends and the heart muscle is at rest, this is called

_____.

15. What electrical activity of the heart is indicated by the P wave?

16. What electrical activity of the heart is indicated by the T wave?

17. Why would a physician order a Holter monitor test?

18. What are some of the conditions that a Doppler study can identify?

Exercise 3

 Online Activity—Preparing for the Electrocardiogram

 30 minutes

1. On the diagram below, identify the locations of the leads to be placed for obtaining an electrocardiograph.

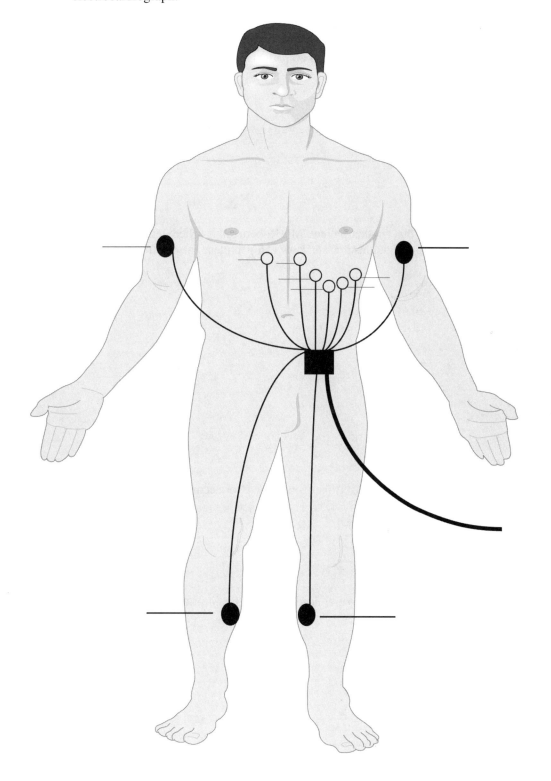

2. If Dr. Simmons had a limb amputation or a bandage or cast on one of his extremities, how would the ECG lead be placed?

3. How should electrodes be placed on patients who have lesions, wounds, or incisions on the chest?

4. Let's assume that another patient, Ms. Robertson, is scheduled to have an ECG. She is obese and has pendulous breasts. How can you place the electrodes on this patient?

5. What clothing should Ms. Robertson remove for accurate placement of the electrodes?

6. What is a rhythm strip? Which lead provides this information?

- Sign in to Mountain View Clinic.
- From the patient list, select **John R. Simmons**.

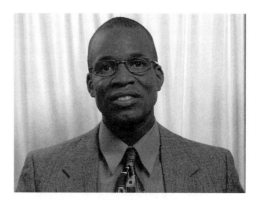

- On the office map, highlight and click on **Exam Room** to enter the examination area.

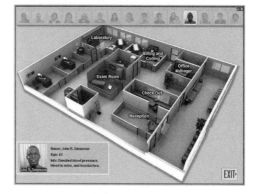

- Under the Watch heading, select **ECG Testing** to begin viewing the video. Pause the video at the first fade-out by clicking the control button on the far left.

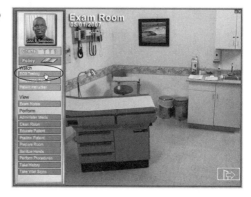

7. Describe Dr. Simmons' position on the table and how he is dressed. Based on this, do you think that he has been appropriately prepared for the ECG?

8. Is it always necessary to remove the patient's shoes and socks when performing an ECG? Why or why not?

9. Dr. Simmons asked Danielle, the medical assisting extern, whether everything was correct. He also stated that his hand was itching during the ECG. Why do you think Dr. Simmons tried to offer a reason for there being a problem with the ECG?

10. Imagine that you were the patient. What reaction do you think you would have if you saw such a perplexed look on the medical assisting extern's face?

11. Danielle then stated that the recording was "fuzzy." What are fuzzy lines on the electro-cardiograph called? What causes these lines?

12. What steps did Danielle take to correct this problem? What other steps could have been taken if her initial attempts had not corrected the problem?

13. Why is it important for Danielle to be sure the abnormal tracing is an artifact rather than a dysrhythmia?

 • Return to the video. Click the play button to continue watching. As you observe the video, consider whether you think Danielle acts professionally.

• Once again, pause the video at the next fade-out.

14. Do you think Danielle acted in a professional manner when discussing the ECG tracing with Dr. Simmons? Explain your answer.

 • Click the play button and watch the remainder of the video.

15. Do you feel that the medical assistant correctly handled the fact that Danielle had discussed the ECG tracing with Dr. Simmons? Explain your answer.

16. On the blank Progress Notes below, document obtaining the electrocardiograph on Dr. Simmons. Use today's date and time for the documentation.

PATIENT'S NAME	☐ FEMALE ☐ MALE Date of Birth: ___/___/___
DATE	PATIENT VISITS AND FINDINGS

ALLERGIC TO _____

_____ PAGE_____ of_____

Urinalysis

Patient: Janet Jones

Learning Objectives:

- Discuss the reasons for performing urinalysis.
- Identify the most common methods of collecting urine specimens in the physician's office.
- Understand the differences in testing results that can be expected with random and clean-catch midstream specimens.
- Identify the guidelines for using reagent strips in performing urinalysis.
- Identify the components of urine.
- Prepare a laboratory requisition for a dipstick urinalysis.
- Differentiate between reliability and accuracy of quality control.
- Identify examples of toxins that can be identified in urine.
- List instructions to be given to a patient who will be collecting a 24-hour urine specimen.
- Document urinalysis results correctly.
- Correlate urine characteristics of a patient with diabetes.

Overview:

This lesson is designed to reinforce the proper procedures for obtaining a clean-catch midstream urine specimen and then performing physical and chemical urinalyses. Janet Jones has a history of kidney disease and will need a urinalysis to provide a differential diagnosis for her back pain. As the medical assistant, you will be expected to understand the necessary information to perform a urinalysis, ensuring quality control.

Exercise 1

Writing Activity—Urine Components and Collection

  25 minutes

1. On the diagram below, label the organs of the urinary tract.

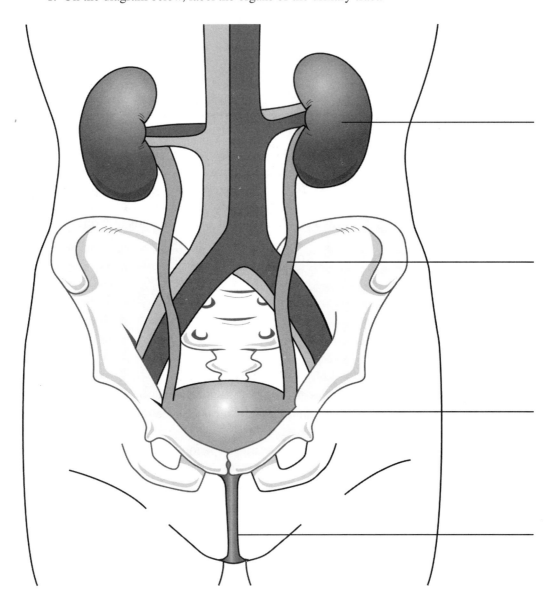

2. Valid reasons for performing urinalyses include which of the following?
   a. For the assessment of pathological conditions in body systems
   b. As a screening measure for the possibility of pathological conditions
   c. To assist in the evaluation of the effectiveness of medical treatment
   d. For the detection of abused substances
   e. All of the above

3. Which of the following are urine collection methods tested routinely in the medical office? Select all that apply.

_____ Random samples

_____ Last-voided specimen of the day

_____ 24-hour urine specimens

_____ Clean-catch midstream specimen

_____ Catheterized specimens

_____ Early-morning voided specimens

_____ First-voided morning specimens

_____ Sterile specimens

4. Which of the following are important guidelines in collecting a urine specimen? Select all that apply.

_____ Obtain a full cup of urine.

_____ Obtain 12-50 mL of urine, with 50 mL being the ideal volume.

_____ Label the specimen with the patient's name only.

_____ Label the specimen with the patient's name and the date and time of collection.

_____ Label the specimen with the patient's name, the date and time of collection, and the type of specimen.

_____ Label the specimen with the patient's name, the date and time of collection, and the initials of the person handling the specimen.

_____ Medications should be recorded on the laboratory requisition.

_____ Collection of urine should be avoided during menstruation.

_____ The medical assistant should allow time for the patient to void and supply water for the patient to drink if necessary.

_____ The medical assistant should not allow the patient to leave the office until the specimen has been collected.

5. What instructions should be given to the patient for a 24-hour urine specimen?

Exercise 2

Online Activity—Performing a Urinalysis

 25 minutes

1. What differences in test results could be expected with random catch and clean-catch midstream urine specimens?

 • Sign in to Mountain View Clinic.
  • From the patient list, select **Janet Jones**.

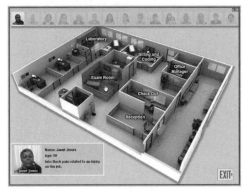

  • On the office map, highlight and click on **Exam Room**.

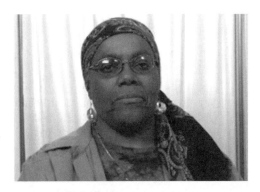

  • Under the Watch heading, select **Specimen Collection** to view the video.

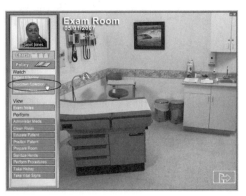

- At the end of the video, click **Close**. Then click on the exit arrow to go to the Summary Menu.
- Click on **Return to Map**.
- From the office map, highlight and click on **Billing and Coding**.

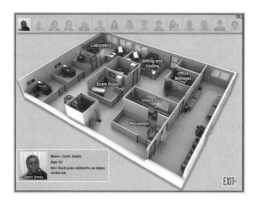

- Click on **Charts** to open Ms. Jones' medical record.

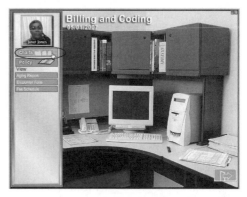

- When the chart opens, click on the **Consultation & Referral** tab. Then select **2-Progress Notes** from the drop-down menu.
- Review Ms. Jones' Progress Notes, specifically watching for data regarding her previous medical history.

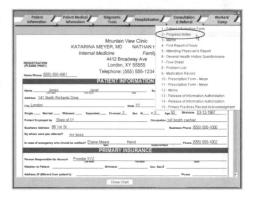

2. Why would it be important for Ms. Jones to provide a urine specimen based on her medical history?

3. What is ureterolithiasis?

4. The three components of a urinalysis are _____,

   _____, and _____ analysis of the urine.

5. In a urinalysis, what four physical properties should be determined?

6. Which of the following are valid labels for the appearance of urine?

   _____ Clear

   _____ Smokey

   _____ Bright

   _____ Cloudy

   _____ Turbid (very cloudy)

   _____ OK

   _____ Hazy

7. Which of the following are incorrect words for labeling the color of urine?

   _____ Straw

   _____ Yellow

   _____ Light and dark straw

   _____ Brownish red

   _____ Amber

8. What are some of the causes of odoriferous urine?

9. Urine should have a slightly _____ odor.

10. Indicate whether each of the following statements is true or false.

    a. _____ Cloudiness of urine is always a sign that the urine contains bacteria.

    b. _____ Urine should be tested as soon as possible after collection.

    c. _____ The smell of ammonia may be an indication of a UTI due to bacterial action.

    d. _____ The color of urine is determined by the concentration of urochrome from the breakdown of hemoglobin.

    e. _____ The presence of myoglobin from a muscle crush injury cannot be distinguished from hemoglobinuria with dipstick testing.

    f. _____ Blood is always visually apparent in urine when present.

    g. _____ A fruity odor to urine may be a sign of diabetes.

    h. _____ The longer urine stands after collection, the more likely bacteria are to grow at room temperature.

    i. _____ Morphine, methadone, PCP, tricyclics, marijuana, Ecstasy, and methamphetamines are toxins that may be identified in a patient's urine by performing a rapid drug screen.

11. Do you think that the medical assistant in the video was professional in providing information to Ms. Jones? Support your answer.

12. _____ (**Reliability** or **Accuracy**) refers to how close the obtained value of a test result is to the real true value.

13. _____ (**Reliability** or **Accuracy**) refers to the reproducibility of a test procedure.

14. Which of the following can be found on a dipstick urine test? Select all that apply.

    _____ Protein

    _____ Alcohol

    _____ Blood

    _____ Leukocyte esterase

    _____ Glucose

    _____ Ketones

_____ Urobilinogen

_____ Bile

_____ Bilirubin

_____ Nitrite

_____ pH

_____ Specific gravity

_____ Color

15. Which of the following are proper guidelines for using reagent strips for urine testing? Select all that apply.

_____ The specimen should be freshly voided.

_____ Reagent strips may be used only with a clean-catch midstream specimen.

_____ The specimen container should be clean and dry.

_____ The container should be free of detergent.

_____ The container must be sterile.

_____ First-voided morning specimens are concentrated and provide the best results for nitrite and protein determination, bacterial culture, pregnancy testing, and microscopic examination.

_____ Specimens should be read against the color card for the test.

_____ The amount of lighting available when reading the test is not important.

_____ Reagent strips may be stored under any conditions.

_____ The desiccant in the specimen bottle should remain in place until all strips have been used.

_____ Reagent strips are best when stored in the refrigerator.

_____ Discoloration of the strips has no effect on testing.

_____ Quality control on the strips should be performed each day.

_____ Quality control ensures reliability of the test results.

16. Indicate whether each of the following statements concerning microscopic examination of specimens is true or false.

a. _____ Microscopic examination of urine specimens is a CLIA-waived test.

b. _____ Red blood cells in urine are easily seen under a microscope.

c. _____ White blood cells are larger than red blood cells and are more easily seen.

d. _____ Epithelial cells in urine are the result of sloughing of the outer layer of skin.

e. _____ Squamous epithelial cells are not uncommon in urine specimens of females.

f. _____ Renal epithelial cells are considered normal in a urine specimen.

g. _____ Various crystals and casts may be found in urine.

h. _____ Drugs may produce crystals in urine.

i. _____ If urine is left to sit out or becomes cold, crystals may precipitate.

17. On the blank Progress Notes below, document the urine specimen testing results for Janet Jones (using today's date and time). Include color (amber) and turbidity (cloudy). The dipstick urine results are as follows: albumin 1+; glucose 3+; leukocytes moderate.

PATIENT'S NAME	☐ FEMALE ☐ MALE Date of Birth: __/__/__
DATE	PATIENT VISITS AND FINDINGS

ALLERGIC TO _____

PAGE _____ of _____

18. If Dr. Meyer believed it was necessary, she could have ordered a random urine specimen for Ms. Jones to be sent to the laboratory for routine urinalysis with a microscopic analysis. Prepare the laboratory requisition form below to order this test for the patient (using today's date and the time of her appointment).

Lab Services

IMPORTANT
Patient instructions and map on back

PHYSICIAN ORDERS

Patient _____ Last Name _____ First _____ M.I.   M ☐ Patient   D.O.B. _____ F ☐   SS# ___ – ___ – ___

Address _____ City _____ Zip _____ Phone # _____

Physician _____
ATTACH COPY OF INSURANCE CARD

Date & Time of Collection: _____ _____
Drawing Facility:

Diagnosis/ICD-9 Code _____
(Additional codes on reverse)

☐ ROUTINE   ☐ PHONE RESULTS TO: # _____
☐ ASAP   ☐ FAX RESULTS TO: # _____
☐ STAT   ☐ COPY TO: _____

☐ 789.00 Abdominal Pain ☐ 414.9 Coronary Artery Disease (CAD) ☐ 244.9 Hypothyroidism
☐ 285.9 Anemia (NOS) ☐ 250.0 DM (diabetes mellitus) ☐ 272.4 Hyperlipidemia
☐ 780.7 Fatigue/Malaise ☐ 401.9 Hypertension
☐ 272.0 Hypercholesterolemia ☐ 485.9 URI (upper respiratory infection)

HEMATOLOGY
☐ 1021 CBC, Automated Diff (incl. Platelet Ct.)
☐ 1023 Hemoglobin/Hematocrit
☐ 1020 Hemogram
☐ 1025 Platelet Count
☐ 1150 Pro Time Diagnostic
☐ 1151 Pro Time, Therapeutic
☐ 1155 PTT
☐ 1315 Reticulocyte Count
☐ 1310 Sed Rate/Westergren

URINE
☐ 1059 Urinalysis
☐ 1082 Urinalysis w/Culture if indicated
Urine-24 Hr ____ Spot ____
Ht. ____ Wt. ____
☐ 3033 Creatinine
☐ 3036 Creatinine Clearance (also requires blood)
☐ 3398 Protein
☐ 3096 Sodium/Potassium
☐ Microalbumin 24 Hr ____ Spot ____

SEROLOGY
☐ 8020 ANA (Antinuclear Antibody)
☐ 8040 Mono Spot
☐ 3494 Rheumatoid Factor
☐ 8010 RPR
☐ 5365 Rubella

CHEMISTRY
☐ 5550 Alpha Fetoprotein, Prenatal
☐ 3000 Amylase
☐ 3153 B12/Folate
☐ 3156 Beta HCG, Quantitative
☐ 3321 Bilirubin, Total
☐ 3324 Bilirubin, Total/Direct
☐ 3009 BUN
☐ 3159 CEA
☐ 3348 Cholesterol
☐ 3030 Creatinine, Serum
☐ 3509 Digoxin (recommend 12 hrs. after dose)
☐ 3515 Dilantin
☐ 3168 Ferritin
☐ 3193 FSH
☐ 3066 ▼ Glucose, Fasting
☐ 3061 Glucose, 1° Post 50 g Glucola
☐ 3075 ▼ Glucose, 2° Post Glucola
☐ 3060 Glucose, 2° Post Prandial (meal)
☐ 3049 ▼ Glucose Tolerance Oral GTT
☐ 3047 ▼Glucose Tolerance Gestational GTT
☐ 3650 Hemoglobin, A1C

CHEMISTRY
☐ 5232 HBsAg
☐ 3175 HIV (Consent required)
☐ 3581 Iron & Iron Binding Capacity
☐ 3195 LH
☐ 3590 Magnesium
☐ 3527 Phenobarbital
☐ 3095 Potassium
☐ 3689 Pregnancy Test, Serum (HCG, qual)
☐ 3653 Pregnancy Test, Urine
☐ 3197 Prolactin
☐ 3199 PSA
☐ 3339 SGOT/AST
☐ 3342 SGPT/ALT
☐ 3093 Sodium/Potassium, Serum
☐ 3510 Tegretol
☐ 3551 Theophylline
☐ 3333 Uric Acid

MICROBIOLOGY
Source _____
☐ 7240 Culture, AFB
☐ 7200 Culture, Blood x ____
☐ Draw Interval ____
☐ 7280 Culture, Fungus
☐ Culture, Routine
☐ 7005 Culture, Stool
☐ 7010 Culture, Throat
☐ 7000 Culture, Urine
☐ 7300 Gram Stain
☐ 7355 Occult Blood x ____
☐ 7365 Ova & Parasites x ____
☐ 7400 Smear & Suspension
(includes Gram Stain/Wet Mount)
☐ 7060 Rapid Strep A Screen (Negs confir by cult)
☐ 7065 Rapid Strep A Screen only
☐ 7030 Beta Strep Culture
☐ 5207 GC by DNA Probe
☐ 5130 Chlamydia by DNA Probe
☐ 5555 Chlamydia/GC by DNA Probe
☐ 7375 Wright Stain, Stool

Additional Tests _____

PANELS & PROFILES
☐ ✗ 3309 CHEM 12
Albumin, Alkaline Phosphatase, BUN, Calcium, Cholesterol, Glucose, LDH, Phosphorus, AST, Total Bilirubin, Total Protein, Uric Acid
☐ ▼ 3315 CHEM 20
Chem 12, Electrolyte Panel, Creatinine, Iron, Gamma GT, ALT, Triglycerides
☐ ▼ 3357 CARDIAC RISK PANEL
Cholesterol, HDL, LDL, Risk Factors, VLDL Triglycerides
☐ ✗ 3042 CRITICAL CARE PANEL
BUN, Chloride, CO2, Glucose, Potassium, Sodium
☐ 3046 ELECTROLYTE PANEL
Chloride, CO2, Potassium, Sodium
☐ ▼ 3399 EXECUTIVE PANEL
Chem 20, Iron, Cardiac Risk Panel, CBC, RPR, Thyroid Cascade

☐ 5242 HEPATITIS PANEL, ACUTE
HAVIgMAb, HBsAg, HBsAb, HBcAb, HCVAb
☐ ▼ 3355 LIPID MONITORING PANEL
Cholesterol, Triglycerides, HDL, LDL, VLDL, ALT, AST
☐ 3312 LIVER PANEL
Alkaline Phospatase, AST, Total Bilirubin, Gamma GT, Total Protein, Albumin, ALT
☐ ✗ 3083 METABOLIC STATUS PANEL
BUN, Osmolality (calculated), Chloride, CO2, Creatinine, Glucose, Potassium, Sodium, BUN/Creatinine, Ratio, Anion Gap
☐ ✗ 3376 PANEL B
Chem 12, CBC, Electrolyte Panel
☐ ▼ 3382 PANEL D
Chem 20, CBC, Thyroid Cascade
☐ ✗ 3388 PANEL F
Chem 12, CBC, Electrolyte Panel, Thyroid Cascade

☐ ▼ 3391 PANEL G
Chem 20, Cardiac Risk Panel, CBC, Thyroid Cascade
☐ ▼ 3393 PANEL H
Chem 20, CBC, Cardiac Risk Panel, Rheumatoid Factor, Thyroid Cascade
☐ ▼ 3397 PANEL J
Chem 20, Cardiac Risk Panel
☐ 5351 PRENATAL PANEL
Antibody Screen ABO/Rh, CBC, Rubella, HBsAg, RPR
☐ 1059 with Urinalysis, Routine
☐ 1082 with Urinalysis w/Culture if Indicated
☐ ✗ 3102 RENAL PANEL
Metabolic Status Panel, Calcium, Phosphorus
☐ 3188 THYROID CASCADE
TSH, Reflex Testing

▼ - patient **required** to fast for 12-14 hours
✗ - patient recommended to fast 12-14 hours

LAB USE ONLY
☐ SST ☐ PLASMA
☐ PURPLE ☐ SERUM
☐ YELLOW ☐ SWAB
☐ BLUE ☐ SLIDES
☐ GREEN ☐ DNA PROBE
☐ GREY ☐ B. CULT BTLS
☐ URINE
☐ BLACK
☐ OTHER: ____
REC'V. SPECIMEN: ☐ FROZEN
☐ AMBIENT ☐ ON ICE
INIT ____

Special Instructions/Pertinent Clinical Information _____

Physician's Signature _____   Date _____
These orders may be FAXed to: 449-5288

7060-500 (7/96)

LAB

Critical Thinking Question

19. If a patient is injured on the job, as was Ms. Jones, would you expect the employer to request a urine toxicology or drug screen on the employee after the injury occurred? Why or why not?

Collecting Urine Specimens

Reading Assignment: Chapter 52—Assisting in the Analysis of Urine
- Collecting a Urine Specimen

Patient: Louise Parlet

Learning Objectives:

- Discuss the reason for giving appropriate instructions to the patient before obtaining clean-catch midstream urine specimens.
- Identify the correct order of the steps needed to prepare a patient, either male or female, for obtaining a clean-catch midstream urine specimen.
- Discuss how breaks in proper technique can lead to possible errors in diagnoses.
- Distinguish between correct and incorrect instructions for collecting a urine specimen.
- Complete a laboratory requisition form for a urine specimen.
- Understand the time limit for allowing urine to sit at room temperature before specimen integrity is compromised.

Overview:

Clean-catch midstream urine specimens are routinely obtained from patients for analysis for chemicals and possible bacteria. Because urinary catheterization is an invasive procedure, contamination by bacteria can be a problem. The clean-catch midstream procedure is the most effective means of obtaining a specimen that is as free of bacteria as possible. However, for the specimen to be of acceptable quality for examination, the patient must be given clear and specific instructions for collection. This lesson will focus on the medical assistant's role in providing patient education and ensuring the necessary steps for quality collection of a clean-catch midstream urine sample.

Exercise 1

 Online Activity—Patient Education for
                        Clean-Catch Midstream Urine Collection

🕐 30 minutes

1. Why is it so important to provide proper patient education about the correct collection method for obtaining a clean-catch midstream urine specimen?

2. Indicate whether each of the following statements is true or false.

   a. _____ All urine specimens collected in the medical office must be clean-catch midstream samples.

   b. _____ The container used to obtain a clean-catch midstream urine sample must be aseptically clean.

   c. _____ The clean-catch midstream procedure requires the patient to follow specific instructions when obtaining the specimen.

   d. _____ A clean-catch midstream urine sample is used to check for urinary tract infections.

   e. _____ The patient has responsibility in the proper collection of the specimen.

   f. _____ Before collecting the specimen, a female patient should cleanse the perineum from back to front.

   g. _____ Before collecting the specimen, a male patient should cleanse the head of the penis in a circular motion from the urethral opening outward.

 • Sign in to Mountain View Clinic.
   • Select **Louise Parlet** from the patient list.

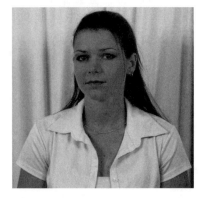

➤ • On the office map, click on **Exam Room**.

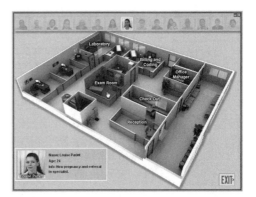

• Under the Watch heading, select **Urine Specimen Collection** to view the video.

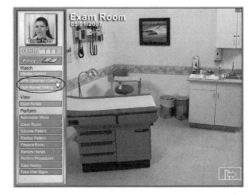

3. In the video, the medical assistant provided incorrect information. What incorrect information was given to the patient? What would be the correct instruction?

➤ • Next, under the Perform heading, click on **Prepare Room**.

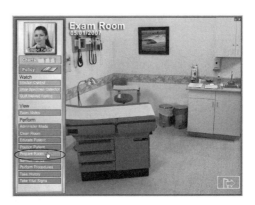

- Begin choosing the supplies needed for Louise Parlet's visit. (*Note:* You can open the patient's Exam Notes for reference as you make your selections.)
- Continue selecting supplies until you are satisfied you have everything you need from the list.
- After completing your selections, click **Finish** to return to the Exam Room.
- Click the exit arrow to go to the Summary Menu.

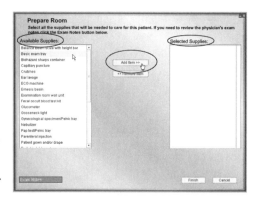

- Click on **Look at Your Performance Summary**. Scroll down to the Prepare Room section to compare your answers with those of the experts. This summary can also be printed or saved for your instructor.
- Click on **Close** to return to the Summary Menu.
- Click on **Return to Map**.

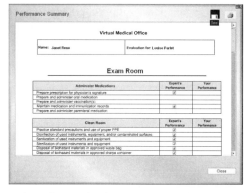

4. Match the following columns to show the correct order of steps in the collection of a clean-catch midstream urine specimen for a female patient.

Order	Action
_____ Step 1	a. Wipe, redress, wash your hands, and return urine to the place designated.
_____ Step 2	
_____ Step 3	b. Wash your hands and open the towelette packages for easy access.
_____ Step 4	c. Cleanse each side of the urinary meatus with a front-to-back motion from the pubis to the anus, using a separate antiseptic wipe to clean each side. Clean directly across the urinary meatus with a third wipe.
_____ Step 5	
_____ Step 6	d. Complete voiding into the toilet.
_____ Step 7	e. Void a small amount of urine, not catching the urine in the container.
_____ Step 8	f. Void into the container.
_____ Step 9	g. Move the container into position to catch the urine.
_____ Step 10	h. Remove undergarment, sit on the toilet swinging one leg to the side, and expose the urinary meatus by spreading apart the labia with one hand.
	i. Open the collection container without touching the rim or inside and place the lid facing up on a paper towel.
	j. Close the container, taking care not to touch the rim or inside.

5. Why is it important that the patient be reminded to wash his or her hands before obtaining the specimen?

6. What are some of the possible problems that may be encountered if the patient is not properly prepared for obtaining the urine specimen?

7. After the specimen has been collected, how long should it be allowed to stand prior to testing?

8. Which of the following should be included in charting the collection of a clean-catch midstream urine specimen? Select all that apply.

_____ Date of collection

_____ Time of collection

_____ Time that the specimen was provided to the laboratory

_____ Type of specimen collected

_____ Instructions provided to the patient

_____ Type of test ordered

_____ Signature of person doing the charting

→ • On the office map, highlight and click on **Laboratory**.

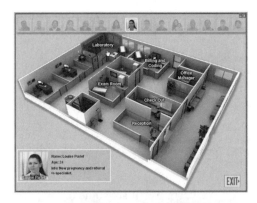

• Under the Perform heading, click on **Collect Specimens**.
• Next, select all the tests ordered for Louise Parlet that require urine collection. (*Note:* If you wish to review the notes for this visit, click on **Charts** and select **3-Progress Notes** from the menu under the **Patient Medical Information** tab.)
• A series of questions will be asked for each test you selected. Answer all the questions related to each test; then click **Finish** to return to the Laboratory. (*Remember:* The Policy Manual can be opened at any time for reference as you answer the questions.)
• Click on **Charts** and then on the **Patient Medical Information** tab. Select **3-Progress Notes** from the drop-down menu.

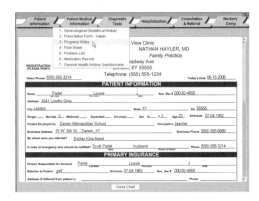

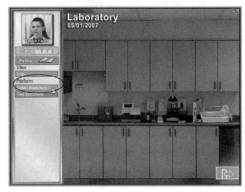

9. Below, complete the laboratory requisition form as ordered in the Progress Notes by Dr. Hayler.

Lab Services

IMPORTANT
Patient instructions
and map on back

PHYSICIAN ORDERS

M ☐ Patient

Patient _____ _____ _____ D.O.B. _____ F ☐ SS# ___ – ___ – ___
　　　　　Last Name　　　　　　　　　First　　　　　　　　M.I.

Address _____ City _____ Zip _____ Phone # _____

Physician _____
ATTACH COPY OF INSURANCE CARD

Date & Time of Collection:
_____
_____

Drawing
Facility: _____

Diagnosis/ICD-9 Code _____
(Additional codes on reverse)

☐ ROUTINE　☐ PHONE RESULTS TO: # _____

☐ 789.00 Abdominal Pain　☐ 414.9 Coronary Artery Disease (CAD)　☐ 244.9 Hypothyroidism
☐ 285.9 Anemia (NOS)　☐ 250.0 DM (diabetes mellitus)　☐ 272.4 Hyperlipidemia
☐ 780.7 Fatigue/Malaise　☐ 401.9 Hypertension
☐ 272.0 Hypercholesterolemia　☐ 485.9 URI (upper respiratory infection)

☐ ASAP　☐ FAX RESULTS TO: # _____

☐ STAT　☐ COPY TO: _____

HEMATOLOGY	CHEMISTRY	CHEMISTRY	MICROBIOLOGY
☐ 1021 CBC, Automated Diff (incl. Platelet Ct.)	☐ 5550 Alpha Fetoprotein, Prenatal	☐ 5232 HBsAg	Source _____
☐ 1023 Hemoglobin/Hematocrit	☐ 3000 Amylase	☐ 3175 HIV (Consent required)	☐ 7240 Culture, AFB
☐ 1020 Hemogram	☐ 3153 B12/Folate	☐ 3581 Iron & Iron Binding Capacity	☐ 7200 Culture, Blood x _____
☐ 1025 Platelet Count	☐ 3156 Beta HCG, Quantitative	☐ 3195 LH	☐ Draw Interval _____
☐ 1150 Pro Time Diagnostic	☐ 3321 Bilirubin, Total	☐ 3590 Magnesium	☐ 7280 Culture, Fungus
☐ 1151 Pro Time, Therapeutic	☐ 3324 Bilirubin, Total/Direct	☐ 3527 Phenobarbital	☐ Culture, Routine
☐ 1155 PTT	☐ 3009 BUN	☐ 3095 Potassium	☐ 7005 Culture, Stool
☐ 1315 Reticulocyte Count	☐ 3159 CEA	☐ 3689 Pregnancy Test, Serum (HCG, qual)	☐ 7010 Culture, Throat
☐ 1310 Sed Rate/Westergren	☐ 3348 Cholesterol	☐ 3653 Pregnancy Test, Urine	☐ 7000 Culture, Urine
	☐ 3030 Creatinine, Serum	☐ 3197 Prolactin	☐ 7300 Gram Stain
URINE	☐ 3509 Digoxin (recommend 12 hrs., after dose)	☐ 3199 PSA	☐ 7355 Occult Blood x _____
☐ 1059 Urinalysis	☐ 3515 Dilantin	☐ 3339 SGOT/AST	☐ 7365 Ova & Parasites x _____
☐ 1082 Urinalysis w/Culture if indicated	☐ 3168 Ferritin	☐ 3342 SGPT/ALT	☐ 7400 Smear & Suspension
Urine-24 Hr _____ Spot _____	☐ 3193 FSH	☐ 3093 Sodium/Potassium, Serum	(includes Gram Stain/Wet Mount)
Ht. _____ Wt. _____	☐ 3066 ▼ Glucose, Fasting	☐ 3510 Tegretol	☐ 7060 Rapid Strep A Screen (Negs confir by cult)
☐ 3033 Creatinine	☐ 3061 Glucose, 1° Post 50 g Glucola	☐ 3551 Theophylline	☐ 7065 Rapid Strep A Screen only
☐ 3036 Creatinine Clearance (also requires blood)	☐ 3075 ▼ Glucose, 2° Post Glucola	☐ 3333 Uric Acid	☐ 7030 Beta Strep Culture
☐ 3398 Protein	☐ 3060 Glucose, 2° Post Prandial (meal)		☐ 5207 GC by DNA Probe
☐ 3096 Sodium/Potassium	☐ 3049 ▼ Glucose Tolerance Oral GTT		☐ 5130 Chlamydia by DNA Probe
☐ Microalbumin 24 Hr _____ Spot _____	☐ 3047 ▼ Glucose Tolerance Gestational GTT		☐ 5555 Chlamydia/GC by DNA Probe
	☐ 3650 Hemoglobin, A1C		☐ 7375 Wright Stain, Stool
SEROLOGY			
☐ 8020 ANA (Antinuclear Antibody)			
☐ 8040 Mono Spot			
☐ 3494 Rheumatoid Factor			
☐ 8010 RPR			
☐ 5365 Rubella	Additional Tests _____		

PANELS & PROFILES

☐ ✗ **3309 CHEM 12**
Albumin, Alkaline Phosphatase, BUN, Calcium, Cholesterol, Glucose, LDH, Phosphorus, AST, Total Bilirubin, Total Protein, Uric Acid

☐ ▼ **3315 CHEM 20**
Chem 12, Electrolyte Panel, Creatinine, Iron, Gamma GT, ALT, Triglycerides

☐ ▼ **3357 CARDIAC RISK PANEL**
Cholesterol, HDL, LDL, Risk Factors, VLDL Triglycerides

☐ ✗ **3042 CRITICAL CARE PANEL**
BUN, Chloride, CO2, Glucose, Potassium, Sodium

☐ **3046 ELECTROLYTE PANEL**
Chloride, CO2, Potassium, Sodium

☐ ▼ **3399 EXECUTIVE PANEL**
Chem 20, Iron, Cardiac Risk Panel, CBC, RPR, Thyroid Cascade

☐ **5242 HEPATITIS PANEL, ACUTE**
HAVIgMAb, HBsAg, HBsAb, HBcAb, HCVAb

☐ ▼ **3355 LIPID MONITORING PANEL**
Cholesterol, Triglycerides, HDL, LDL, VLDL, ALT, AST

☐ **3312 LIVER PANEL**
Alkaline Phosphatase, AST, Total Bilirubin, Gamma GT, Total Protein, Albumin, ALT

☐ ✗ **3083 METABOLIC STATUS PANEL**
BUN, Osmolality (calculated), Chloride, CO2 Creatinine, Glucose, Potassium, Sodium, BUN/Creatinine, Ratio, Anion Gap

☐ ✗ **3376 PANEL B**
Chem 12, CBC, Electrolyte Panel

☐ ▼ **3382 PANEL D**
Chem 20, CBC, Thyroid Cascade

☐ ✗ **3388 PANEL F**
Chem 12, CBC, Electrolyte Panel, Thyroid Cascade

☐ ▼ **3391 PANEL G**
Chem 20, Cardiac Risk Panel, CBC, Thyroid Cascade

☐ ▼ **3393 PANEL H**
Chem 20, CBC, Cardiac Risk Panel, Rheumatoid Factor, Thyroid Cascade

☐ ▼ **3397 PANEL J**
Chem 20, Cardiac Risk Panel

☐ **5351 PRENATAL PANEL**
Antibody Screen ABO/Rh, CBC Rubella, HBsAg, RPR
☐ 1059 with Urinalysis, Routine
☐ 1082 with Urinalysis w/Culture if indicated

☐ ✗ **3102 RENAL PANEL**
Metabolic Status Panel, Calcium, Phosphorus

☐ **3188 THYROID CASCADE**
TSH, Reflex Testing

▼ - patient **required** to fast for 12-14 hours

✗ - patient recommended to fast 12-14 hours

LAB USE ONLY		INIT _____
☐ SST	☐ PLASMA	
☐ PURPLE	☐ SERUM	
☐ YELLOW	☐ SWAB	
☐ BLUE	☐ SLIDES	
☐ GREEN	☐ DNA PROBE	
☐ GREY	☐ B. CULT BTLS	
☐ URINE		
☐ BLACK		
☐ OTHER:		
REC'V. SPECIMEN:	☐ FROZEN	
☐ AMBIENT	☐ ON ICE	

Special Instructions/Pertinent Clinical Information _____

Physician's Signature _____　**Date** _____

These orders may be FAXed to: 449-5288

7060-500 (7/96)

LAB

10. Note that a urine culture can be ordered in two different places on the laboratory requisition. What is the difference between the two?

Obtaining Specimens for Microbiological Testing

📖 **Reading Assignment:** Chapter 55—Assisting in Microbiology and Immunology

Patient: Tristan Tsosie

Learning Objectives:

- Discuss the difference between pathogens and nonpathogens.
- Understand the proper procedure for obtaining wound exudate for microbiological testing.
- Identify the correct handling and transportation of a microbiological specimen.
- Discuss the reasons for using appropriate PPE when obtaining microbiological specimens.
- Document the transport of a microbiological specimen in the laboratory log.
- Apply critical thinking skills in answering questions regarding inconsistency in charting examples.

Overview:

In this lesson the information regarding obtaining a throat specimen and a specimen for microbiological testing will be presented. Tristan Tsosie is an 8-year-old boy with a history of injury to his arm. His Exam Notes also indicate he has a sore throat. You will determine the proper care of Tristan to fulfill the orders of the physician. The patient, who is to have suture removal and a cast check, is accompanied by his sister and another child. There are some inconsistencies in this lesson of which you should make a note. The inconsistencies will be addressed with thought questions at the end of the lesson. *Remember:* When accessing the Progress Notes, you have to be in the designated room to see the correct notes.

Exercise 1

Online Activity—Obtaining a Wound Specimen for Microbiological Testing

20 minutes

- Sign in to Mountain View Clinic.
- From the patient list, select **Tristan Tsosie**.
- If you need to refresh your memory from an earlier lesson, you may go to the Reception area and review Tristan's Check-In video.

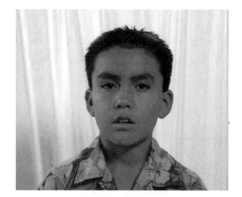

- On the office map, click to enter the **Exam Room**.

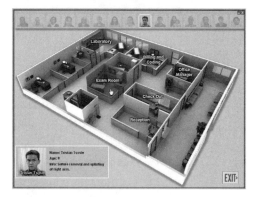

- From the Exam Room menu, select **Wound Care** and watch the video.

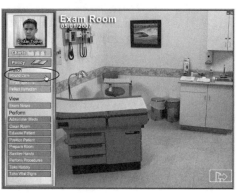

1. In the video, the medical assistant states that a wound specimen for testing will be obtained. Why is the wound specimen being taken from Tristan's arm?

2. Why should the specimen be taken before cleansing the wound?

 • Click **Close** at the end of the video and return to the Exam Room.
• Under Perform, select **Prepare Room** and choose the supplies needed for Tristan's visit.
• Click **Finish** to return to the Exam Room.

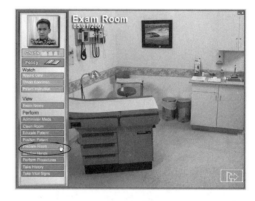

• Next, click on **Exam Notes** to review the initial documentation of Tristan's visit.

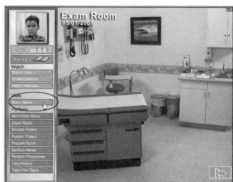

3. What tests have been ordered for Tristan?

 • Click **Finish** to close the Exam Notes.
• Now select **Prepare Room** and choose the supplies and equipment needed for Tristan's examination. Scroll down to that area of the page. (*Note:* If you want to reopen the Exam Notes for reference as you make your selections, click on **Exam Notes** in the bottom left corner of the screen.)
• After completing your selections, click **Finish** to return to the Exam Room.

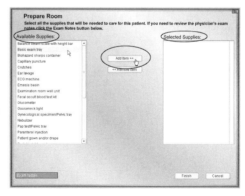

4. Describe the difference between pathogens and nonpathogens. Explain the importance of this in regard to wound care.

5. Indicate whether each of the following statements is true or false.

a. _____ The wound specimen should be taken from the cleanest area of the wound.

b. _____ Wound specimens should be placed in the transport medium immediately after they are obtained.

c. _____ Wound specimens should be dry for transport so that the chance of cross-contamination is reduced.

d. _____ Ideally, wound specimens should be obtained after antibiotic therapy has been initiated.

e. _____ Hands should be sanitized before and after collecting the specimen, even though gloves have been worn.

f. _____ Supplies used in the collection of the wound specimen should be disposed of in the biohazardous waste.

g. _____ Collection of all wound specimens requires the use of gowns and goggles.

h. _____ Collection of the wound specimen is not complete until documentation has been completed.

i. _____ The time between collection of the specimen and the laboratory processing of the specimen is not important.

6. Describe the means used by the medical assistant and the extern to place Tristan at ease during the procedure of collecting the wound specimen.

Thought Question

7. Is there anything that you would have done differently if you were the medical assistant taking care of Tristan?

➤ • From the Exam Room menu, again click on **Exam Notes** to read the documentation concerning the wound.

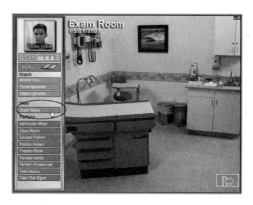

8. Below are the Progress Notes from Tristan's chart showing how the wound specimen collection was documented. Compare this documentation with the Exam Notes. Is there any information that could be, or should be, added to this documentation?

05-01-2007 11:30am	Per radiologist verbally, no change in bone alignment from previous x-ray. Radiographs show non-displaced Colles fracture in first stage of healing. Exam unremarkable except for small amount yellowish drainage visible at proximal edge of well approximated suture line. No obvious inflammation/edema of right arm. Old splint stained and malodorous. Also, oropharynx mildly reddened with small patchy areas of yellowish/white exudate. Negative adenopathy. Denies difficulty swallowing. Reports throat hurts just a little. Afebrile. Impression: Colles fracture in first stage of healing. Wound exudate, possible contamination from dirty splint, R/O wound infection. Mildly inflamed oropharynx, probable URI, R/O strep throat. Plan: Obtain wound culture from right arm. Remove all sutures. Replace contaminated splint with new splint. Do Rapid Strep test. Instruct parent to call in 2 days with update of condition. Follow-up in office in 3 weeks or sooner if develops signs/symptoms of infection or sore throat worsens. Re-educate regarding proper splint care and activity during healing process.--- ---———Nathan Hayler, MD
05-01-2007 11:45am	Wound culture obtained, wound cleaned, 7 stitches removed, and new posterior splint reapplied without apparent intolerance. Appears comfortable, no complaints. Fingers pink and warm. QuickVue In-Line One Step Strep A test done; results negative. Wound culture sent to Quality Lab on 05/01/2007. Given verbal and written instructions on observing for signs of infection, proper splint care, and activity during the healing process. Instructed to have parent call in 2 days with update and to confirm understanding of follow-up care.-- ---———Cathy Wright, CMA/NH
05-01-2007 12:00pm	Mother contacted and given instructions about required follow-up care.--- ---———Leah Tran, CMA/NH

ALLERGIC TO NKA

PAGE 1 of 1

9. **Critical Thinking Question:** Assume the laboratory courier had already picked up the specimens on 5/1/2007. What would be the appropriate measures to take to ensure specimen integrity?

10. How will the medical assistant know the temperature at which to store the specimen until the courier arrives on May 2?

- Click **Finish** and then click on **Policy Manual** to see if there are any notations about what PPE the medical assistant should wear while collecting the throat swab. Remain in the Exam Room with Tristan and continue to Exercise 2.

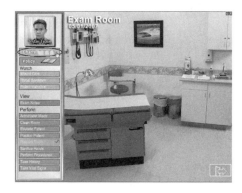

Exercise 2

Online Activity—Collecting a Throat Specimen for Microbiological Testing

 20 minutes

The Policy Manual does not specify the needed protective equipment for a professional who is obtaining a throat specimen; it simply states that OSHA standard precautions should be followed.

1. What protective equipment should be worn by the medical assistant while obtaining a routine throat specimen? When is it necessary to include other PPEs, and what should these be?

- From the Exam Room menu, select **Throat Specimen** and watch the video.

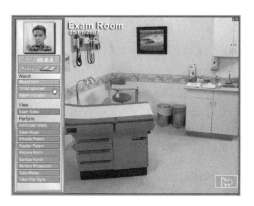

2. What did the medical assistant do to be sure that she had Tristan's cooperation?

- Click the exit arrow to leave the Exam Room.
- On the Summary Menu, click on **Look at Your Performance Summary** to compare your answers with those of the experts.
- Click on **Return to Map**.
- On the office map, click to enter the **Laboratory**.

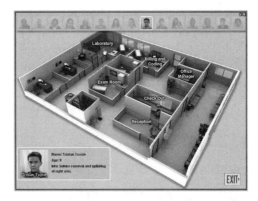

- Under Perform, select **Collect Specimens**.

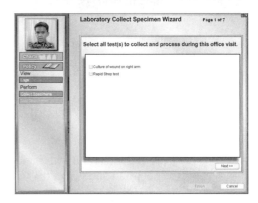

- Next, select the tests ordered for Tristan at this visit. (*Hint:* If you wish to review the notes for the visit, click on **Charts** and select **1-Progress Notes** under **Patient Medical Information**.)
- A series of questions will be asked for *each* test selected. Answer the questions related to each test and click **Finish** to return to the Laboratory. (*Hint:* The Policy Manual can be opened at any time for reference as you answer the questions.)

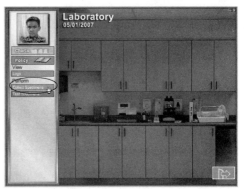

- Click on **Charts**. From the drop-down menu under the **Patient Medical Information** tab select **1-Progress Notes**.

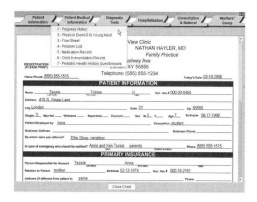

3. What are the results of the strep test that was processed using the specimen?

4. Was the documentation correct for the testing done? Explain your answer.

5. When you are obtaining a throat specimen for testing, what is the most appropriate site for collection?

6. Why would it be advantageous to use two sterile swabs when collecting a specimen? In what situation(s) do you think a specimen would likely be sent to an outside laboratory?

7. Why is it important that the inside of the mouth not be touched while the throat specimen is being obtained?

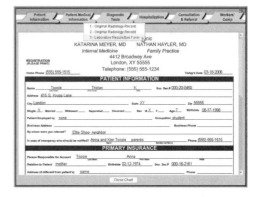

→ • Still in Tristan's chart, click on the **Diagnostic Tests** tab and select **3-Laboratory Requisition Form**.

• Review the Laboratory Requisition Form for accuracy and completeness.

8. Is the Laboratory Requisition Form complete and correct? If not, describe any errors and explain what would need to be done to correct them.

9. What insurance information is to be provided with the requisition?

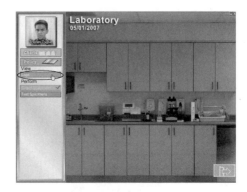

→ • Click **Close Chart** to return to the Laboratory.

• Under View, click on **Logs**.

10. Are all of the tests properly logged for quality control and for following the results of the tests?

 • Click **Finish** to close Lab Log.
 • Click on **Charts** to open Tristan's medical record.
 • Click on the **Patient Medical Information** tab and select **1-Progress Notes** from the drop-down menu.
 • Click **Close Chart** when finished to return to the Billing and Coding area.

11. Earlier in the lesson, what did the Progress Notes say about the date of the transport of the culture to the reference laboratory? (*Hint:* See questions 8 and 9 in Exercise 1.)

12. What do the Progress Notes in the Laboratory say about the date that Tristan's wound culture was sent to the lab?

Thought Question/Critical Thinking

13. Why would it be important to identify discrepancies when charting what happens in the medical office? Does it really matter which date is used?

14. On the blank log below, document the transport of the wound specimen to the laboratory using the 05/01/2007 date. Use the initials "CLW" as the person who collected the specimen.

Requisition Number	Date of Specimen Collected	Patient Name	Laboratory Test	Processing Laboratory	Initials: Specimen Collection	Date of Results Return	Initials: Results Return

- Click **Finish** to return to the Exam Room.
- Select **Look at Your Performance Summary** to compare your answers with those of the experts.
- Expert responses are given separately for each test. Scroll down to locate the test you want to review. Your summary can also be printed or saved for your instructor.
- Click **Close** and select **Return to Map**.

Capillary and Venipuncture Procedures

✐ **Reading Assignment:** Chapter 53—Assisting with Phlebotomy
- Venipuncture Equipment
- Routine Venipuncture
- Problems Associated with Venipuncture
- Specimen Recollection
- Chain of Custody

Patient: Kevin McKinzie

Learning Objectives:

- Identify the most commonly used venipuncture sites.
- Identify the types of specimens that can be obtained by venipuncture.
- Discuss the necessary preparation of the patient for a routine venipuncture.
- Determine what supplies are needed for a venipuncture.
- Review the need for standard precautions with venipuncture.
- Understand why proper positioning of the patient for venipuncture is necessary.
- Identify the process for safe capillary puncture on infants and older children or adults.
- Describe the equipment and supplies needed for capillary puncture.
- Identify methods that can be used to increase blood flow when performing a capillary blood collection.
- Document the collection of blood specimens.
- Indicate how to properly label capillary specimens.

Overview:

In this lesson we will review phlebotomy procedures, including venipuncture and capillary puncture. We will discuss the importance of standard precautions and risk management skills to prevent injury to the patient. Using information obtained from the reading materials, you will analyze proper techniques for venipuncture and capillary puncture, including the proper positioning and education of the patient before the procedure and the proper selection of blood collection tubes for certain types of blood samples. After completing this lesson, you will have an understanding of the different types of blood specimens, as well as the proper disposal of contaminated supplies. We will also address the importance of proper site selection for capillary puncture to reduce discomfort and to ensure the safety of patients, especially infants.

Exercise 1

Online Activity—Identifying the Necessary Supplies for Venipuncture

 25 minutes

- Sign in to Mountain View Clinic.
- Select **Kevin McKinzie** from the patient list.

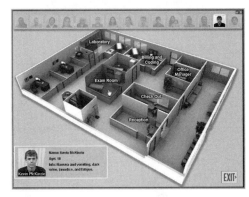

- On the office map, click on **Exam Room**.

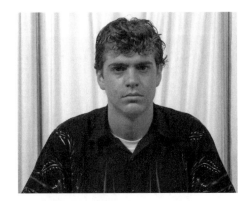

- Select **Exam Notes** to review the notes for the current visit.
- Read the Exam Notes, making note of the blood tests that will require phlebotomy during this visit.
- Click **Finish** to close the Exam Notes.

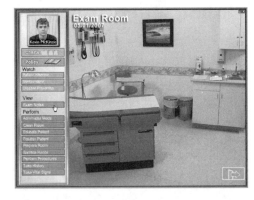

- Now select **Prepare Room** (under Perform) to choose the supplies and equipment needed for Kevin McKinzie's visit.
- From the alphabetical list, select the first item needed for this visit; then click **Add Item** to confirm your choice. The items you select will appear in the Selected Supplies column.
- Repeat this step until you have everything you need from the list. (*Hint:* The Exam Notes are available on the bottom left side of the page if you need to refer to them.)

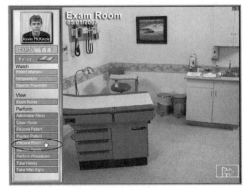

- After completing your selections, click **Finish** to return to the Exam Room.
- Click the exit arrow to go to the Summary Menu.
- Click on **Look at Your Performance Summary**. Scroll down to the Prepare Room section to compare your answers with those of the experts. This summary can be printed or saved for your instructor.
- Click on **Close** and then on **Return to Map**.

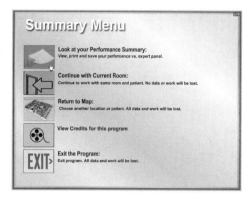

1. Which of the following tests will require blood for completion of the physician's orders for the visit? Select all that apply.

   _____ Urinalysis

   _____ CBC with differential

   _____ Hepatitis panel

   _____ Liver panel

   _____ EBV antibody

   _____ MonoSpot test

2. Which of the tests that you selected in question 1 would be sent to an outside laboratory for testing?

- Using your textbook for reference, decide what types of blood specimens will be needed for the tests ordered.
- On the office map, click to enter the **Laboratory**.

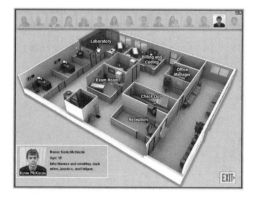

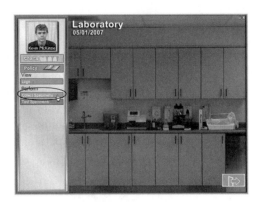

• From the Laboratory menu, under the Perform heading, select **Collect Specimens**.

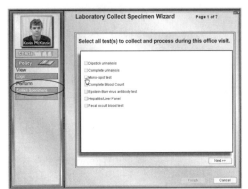

• Next, select all the tests that require blood collection. (*Hint:* If you wish to review the notes for the visit, click on **Charts** and select **1-Progress Notes** under the **Patient Medical Information** tab.)

• A series of questions will be asked for *each* test you selected. Answer all the questions related to each test; then click **Finish** to return to the Laboratory. (*Hint:* The Policy Manual can be opened at any time for reference as you answer the questions.)

• Click the exit arrow to return to the Summary Menu.

• Select **Look at Your Performance Summary** to check your answers against those of the experts.

• Expert responses are given separately for each test. Scroll down to locate the test you want to review. Your summary can be printed or saved for your instructor.

3. Indicate whether each of the following statements is true or false.

   a. _____ Serum is obtained from whole blood that has an anticoagulant added to the test tube to prevent clotting.

   b. _____ Plasma is obtained from whole blood that has an anticoagulant added to the test tube to prevent clotting.

   c. _____ Whole blood is needed for a CBC with differential.

   d. _____ Serum is needed for the hepatitis panel and the liver panel.

   e. _____ Serum contains the chemicals found in the blood with the clotting factors removed.

   f. _____ Plasma contains the chemicals found in the blood with the clotting factors removed.

   g. _____ Evacuated tubes are available in only one size.

   h. _____ Evacuated tubes have an expiration date and a label for writing the patient's name.

i. _____ The evacuated tube may be pushed all the way into the Vacutainer adapter after the needle has entered the vein.

j. _____ If the top of the evacuated tube needs to be opened, a Hemoguard tube should be used.

k. _____ Before using an evacuated tube, you should check it for cracks and other breaches in quality control.

l. _____ If a Vacutainer tube is dropped, it can still be used unless it is cracked or broken.

m. _____ The evacuated tube should be filled to the level of blood specified for the test, not to the size (volume capacity) of the tube.

n. _____ Tubes containing additives should be shaken 8 to 10 times to mix the blood with the additive.

4. Serum can be collected in _____ or _____ tubes that contain no additives.

5. List the parts of the Vacutainer system.

→ • Click on **Close** and then on **Return to Map**.
  • Click on **Exam Room** and continue to Exercise 2.

Exercise 2

Online Activity—Choosing the Correct Position and Site for a Venipuncture

 20 minutes

- In this exercise we will continue with Kevin McKinzie's visit. (*Note:* If you have exited the program, sign in again to Mountain View Clinic, select Kevin McKinzie, and go to the Exam Room.)

1. On the figures below, label the venipuncture sites that are most appropriate for obtaining blood specimens.

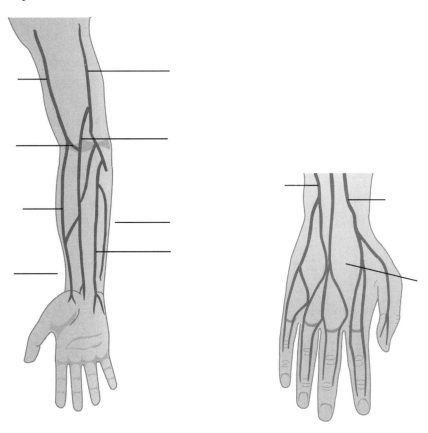

2. What are the advantages of using the veins found in the antecubital area?

3. After applying the tourniquet, if the veins are not easily palpable, what should the next step in venipuncture be?

 • On the office map, click on **Exam Room**.

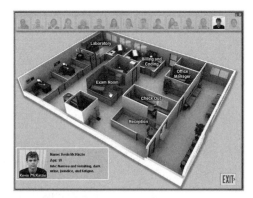

• From the Exam Room menu, select **Venipuncture** and watch the video.
• At the end of the video, click **Close** to return to the Exam Room.

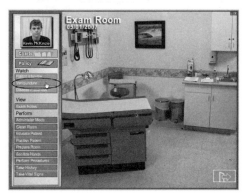

4. What additional steps should have been taken by the medical assistant to make the patient more at ease about the procedure?

5. Why is it important for the patient to be in either a lying or sitting position during venipuncture?

6. Would it ever be appropriate to perform phlebotomy with the patient standing up?

7. Indicate whether each of the following statements is true or false.

   a. _____ Venipuncture may take place on the side of a mastectomy.

   b. _____ Sclerosed veins feel hard and knotty and should not be used for venipuncture.

   c. _____ Veins that are near the top of the skin are always the veins to use for venipuncture.

   d. _____ The angle of the needle for venipuncture is 15 degrees.

   e. _____ When blood is being drawn from the back of the hand, a butterfly needle or winged infusion set is more comfortable and more likely to provide a quality specimen.

   f. _____ The tourniquet should be placed on the arm approximately 4 inches above the venipuncture site when finding the appropriate vein and should remain in place until after the venipuncture is complete, no matter how long the time.

   g. _____ The tourniquet should remain in place until after the needle is removed following venipuncture.

➤ • Remain in the Exam Room with Kevin McKinzie and continue to Exercise 3.

Exercise 3

 Writing Activity—Disposal of Supplies and Handling of Specimen Following Venipuncture

 20 minutes

- Once again, we will continue with Mr. McKinzie's visit. (*Note:* If you have exited the program, sign in again to Mountain View Clinic, select Kevin McKinzie, and go to the Exam Room.)

1. After venipuncture, what is the proper procedure for disposal of the venipuncture supplies?

 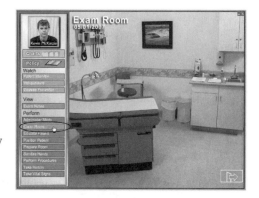

- From the Exam Room menu, click on **Clean Room**.
- Select the appropriate steps to clean the Exam Room after Mr. McKinzie's visit; then click **Finish**.
- Click the exit arrow to return to the Summary Menu.
- Click on **Look at Your Performance Summary** and compare your answers with those of the experts. This summary can be saved or printed for your instructor.
- Click on **Close** and then on **Return to Map**.

2. Indicate whether each of the following statements is true or false.

   a. _____ OSHA has designated that safety-engineered devices on needles should be used to prevent needlestick injuries.

   b. _____ After venipuncture, all materials that have come in contact with the skin must be disposed of in biohazard waste.

   c. _____ OSHA requires that hands be sanitized following venipuncture.

   d. _____ The tourniquet used for the venipuncture should be made of latex and should be sanitized using alcohol so that it may be used for another patient.

   e. _____ Gloves may be removed immediately after the venipuncture, and the test tubes with no gross contamination may be handled without gloves.

   f. _____ Handwashing/hand sanitization should be done after removing gloves and before documentation in the medical record.

g. _____ The length of time a specimen is held following venipuncture and before centrifuging has no significance.

h. _____ Specimens that are not handled with care may have hemolysis.

➤ • On the office map, click on **Laboratory** and then on **Charts**.
  • Click on the **Diagnostic Tests** tab and select **1-Laboratory Requisition Form**.
  • Review the laboratory request to ensure that all tests that are not CLIA-waived have been ordered.

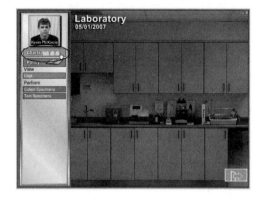

3. Did you find that the tests were correctly ordered?

4. Should any of the tests have been done on the next day because of the need to fast?

➤ • Click **Close Chart** to return to the Laboratory.
  • Now click on **Logs**.

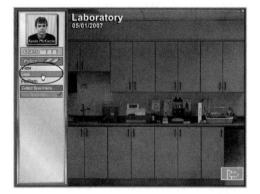

5. Are all of the tests properly logged for quality control and for following the results of the tests?

6. Use the blank log below to document the specimens for Kevin McKinzie as found in the physician's notes.

Requisition Number	Date of Specimen Collected	Patient Name	Laboratory Test	Processing Laboratory	Initials: Specimen Collection	Date of Results Return	Initials: Results Return

Thought Question

7. Why is it unnecessary to include the patient's name and the date on each individual line if multiple tests are being ordered?

 • Click on **Finish** to close the log and return to the Laboratory.
• Under Perform, click on **Test Specimens**.

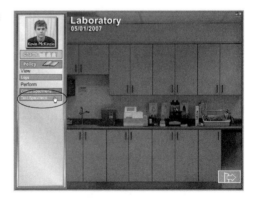

- A series of questions will be asked for *each* test selected. Answer all the questions related to each test and click **Finish** to return to the Laboratory. (*Hint:* The Policy Manual can be opened at any time for reference as you answer the questions.)
- Click on the exit arrow and then on **Return to Map**.
- Remain in the Laboratory with Kevin McKinzie and continue to Exercise 4.

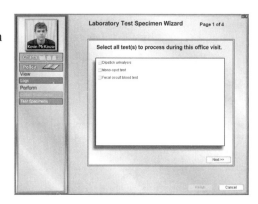

Exercise 4

Online Activity—Documentation of the Specimens

🕐 15 minutes

- Let us continue with Mr. McKinzie's visit. (*Note:* If you have exited the program, sign in again to Mountain View Clinic, select Kevin McKinzie, and go to the Laboratory.)
- Click on **Charts** and then on **Diagnostic Tests**. From the drop-down menu, select **1-Laboratory Requisition Form** and review the tests performed on Mr. McKinzie.

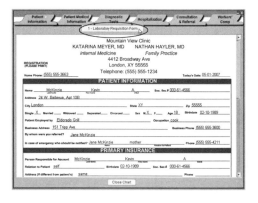

1. Mr. McKinzie's appointment time was 2:45 p.m. Using this information and the tests ordered, document on the blank Progress Notes below the collection of the venipuncture specimens, including the laboratory to which the specimens were sent.

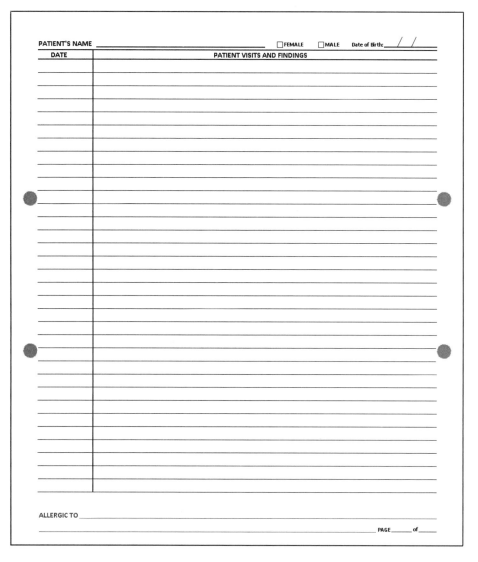

2. What information is lacking from the documentation of the venipuncture in the medical record?

3. What documentation should be placed on the tubes of blood before they are sent to the outside laboratory?

Exercise 5

**Writing Activity—Performing Capillary Puncture on Infants and
Older Children or Adults**

20 minutes

In this exercise you will determine the proper site for capillary puncture for infants and other patients by showing the proper sites on the drawings below. This information will be obtained from your textbook readings.

1. On the figure below, show the proper sites for adult capillary puncture. (*Hint:* Refer to your textbook for this information.)

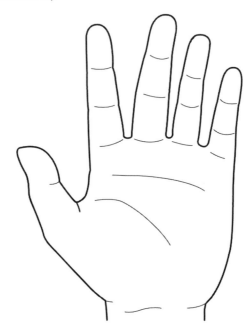

2. On the figure below, show the proper sites for infant capillary puncture. (*Hint:* Refer to your textbook for this information.)

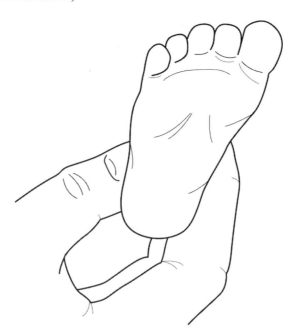

3. List situations in which capillary puncture would be appropriate.

4. Indicate whether each of the following statements is true or false.

a. _____ The site of puncture in an infant is important to prevent the possibility of nerve damage.

b. _____ The site of puncture in an older child or an adult is important to prevent the possibility of nerve damage.

c. _____ The proper selection of a puncture site for an adult is the third or fourth finger of the hand.

d. _____ The length of the lancet to be used for adults and infants is the same.

e. _____ The same collection containers used for venipuncture may be used for capillary punctures.

f. _____ Capillary puncture is used to obtain small amounts of blood.

g. _____ Collection containers for capillary puncture have many of the same additives as those used for venipuncture.

h. _____ The plantar surface of the heel is used for infants who are not yet walking, but this is not the preferred site to use after a child begins walking.

i. _____ All fingers are acceptable sites for capillary puncture.

j. _____ Blood collected with a capillary puncture is pulled into the collection device either by capillary action or by being dropped onto a reagent strip for testing.

k. _____ Documentation of capillary puncture does not necessarily include the site of puncture, but this information should be included for infants.

l. _____ The same safety precautions used with venipuncture should be used with capillary puncture.

m. _____ Because of the added chance of contamination of surfaces by blood, it is wise to have extra supplies such as gloves, gauze pads, and disinfectant readily available.

5. What is the most efficient way to transport capillary tubes?

6. What is one thing you can do to increase blood flow to the area in which you are collecting capillary blood?

LESSON 29

Hematology Testing

/OTO **Reading Assignment:** Chapter 51—Assisting in the Clinical Laboratory
- Role of the Clinical Laboratory in Patient Care

Chapter 53—Assisting in Phlebotomy
- Capillary Puncture

Chapter 54—Assisting in Analysis of Blood
- Hematology
- Collection of Blood Specimens
- Hemoglobin
- Red Blood Cell Count
- White Blood Cell Count
- Red Cell Indices
- Differential Cell Count

Patient: Louise Parlet

Learning Objectives:

- Understand the three levels of laboratory testing as defined by CLIA.
- List the methods for obtaining specimens for CLIA-waived hematology testing.
- Read the Progress Notes correctly.
- List the normal reference range for components of blood that are tested in a complete blood count.
- Discuss the role of the hematology section of the laboratory.
- Describe the collection of blood in a hematocrit tube.
- Explain what is indicated by the MCH, MCV, and MCHC.
- Document laboratory test results on a laboratory flow sheet.

Overview:

In this lesson an understanding of CLIA-waived tests and hematology testing will be emphasized. You will use the Policy Manual to obtain the list of diagnostic tests for a patient with a newly diagnosed pregnancy, Louise Parlet. Finally, you will be expected to add the results of testing to a flow sheet for this patient.

Exercise 1

Online Activity—Performing Diagnostic Tests According to Office Policy

35 minutes

- Sign in to Mountain View Clinic.
- From the patient list, select **Louise Parlet**.

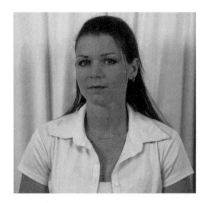

- On the office map, highlight and click on **Exam Room** to enter the examination area.

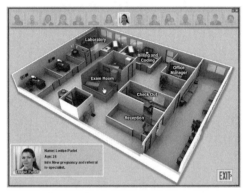

- Under the View heading, click on **Exam Notes** and read the initial documentation of Ms. Parlet's visit.

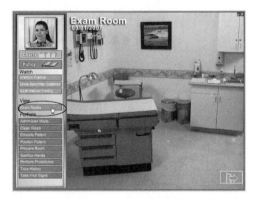

- After reading the Exam Notes, click **Finish** to return to the Exam Room.
- Click on **Policy** to open the Policy Manual.

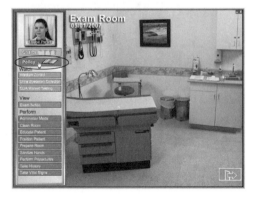

• In the search bar, type "standing orders" and click twice on the magnifying glass to read the section on standing orders, which ends on page 26 of the Policy Manual.

• Leave the Policy Manual open to this page as you answer the following questions.

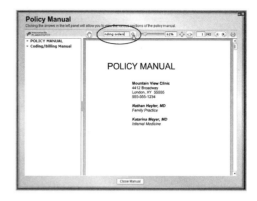

1. What is the primary diagnosis for Ms. Parlet?

2. According to office policy, what tests should be obtained from Ms. Parlet?

 • Click on the arrow next to Policy Manual on the left hand pane to expand the list.

• Click on **Laboratory Policies** to read the laboratory policies.

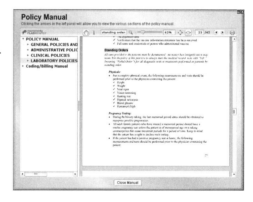

3. What is meant by CLIA?

4. The three levels of CLIA testing are:
   a. simple, moderate, high complexity.
   b. waived, easy, high complexity.
   c. waived, moderate, high complexity.
   d. easy, medium, complex complexity.
   e. waived, medium, complex complexity.

5. Explain "waived tests" as defined by CLIA.

6. List at least four methods for obtaining CLIA-waived tests.

7. Which of the tests you identified in question 2 could be performed as CLIA-waived tests by the medical assistant before the physician sees the patient, since this is the office protocol?

➤ • Click **Close Manual** to return to the Exam Room.
   • Click the exit arrow to go to the Summary Menu.
   • Click **Return to Map**.
   • On the office map, highlight and click on **Billing and Coding**.

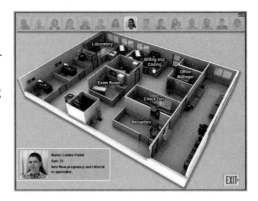

• Click on **Charts**.

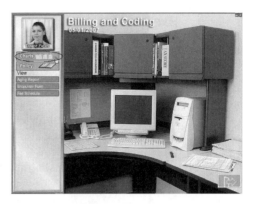

• Next, click on the **Patient Medical Information** tab and select **3-Progress Notes** from the drop-down menu.
• Read the final Progress Notes for Ms. Parlet's visit. Keep the Progress Notes open to complete the remaining exercises.

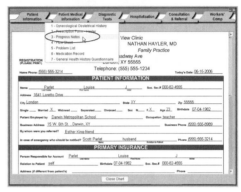

8. According to the Progress Notes, what further blood tests were ordered for Ms. Parlet? Were any of these CLIA-waived?

9. Do the Progress Notes indicate that all the specimens were sent to Quality Lab?

Exercise 2

Writing Activity—Components of Hematology

30 minutes

In this exercise you will review hematology and its components, as well as normal reference ranges for adult patients.

1. Explain the responsibilities of the hematology section of the laboratory.

2. What is the purpose of the "differential count" in the complete blood count (CBC)?

3. Define MCV, MCH, and MCHC.

4. For each blood component listed below, identify the normal range for males and females.

Blood Component	Normal Range by Gender
Red blood cells (erythrocytes)	
White blood cells	
Hemoglobin (Hgb)	
Hematocrit (Hct)	
Platelets	
WBC differential	

5. Describe the collection of a capillary puncture specimen in a calibrated capillary tube for a spun hematocrit.

6. What should the medical assistant do if air bubbles are present in the capillary tube?

7. Why is it important for no air bubbles to be in the capillary puncture specimen for a spun hematocrit?

8. On the diagram below, label the cellular elements found in a capillary tube following centrifuging.

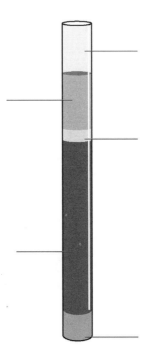

9. When a capillary tube is being spun in a microhematocrit centrifuge, which of the following are necessary for safety? Select all that apply.

_____ PPE

_____ Placing the capillary tube anywhere in the centrifuge

_____ Placing the capillary tubes opposite each other for balance

_____ Placing the sealed edge of the capillary tube toward the exterior of the centrifuge

_____ Placing the capillary tube toward the center of the centrifuge

_____ Closing the lid of the centrifuge before spinning the capillary tube

_____ Opening the lid immediately after the centrifuge stops the cycle

_____ Opening the lid when the centrifuge stops spinning

Exercise 3

Writing Activity—Documenting Hematology Testing

 20 minutes

- In this exercise you will document Louise Parlet's laboratory results in her Progress Notes and on the flow sheet. (*Note:* If you have exited the program, sign in again to Mountain View Clinic, select Louise Parlet, go to the Billing and Coding Room, and click on **Charts**.)

- Under the **Patient Medical Information** tab, select **4-Flow Sheet** and review the flow sheet for today's visit. Remember to scroll down to see the entire flow sheet.

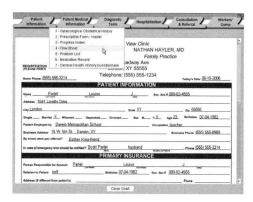

1. The only CLIA-waived test documented for Ms. Parlet was her urine HCG. Her hemoglobin (Hgb), her glucose level, and a dipstick urine were also tested, but they were not documented until after the patient left the office at 9:45 a.m. On the blank Progress Notes below, document the following CLIA-waived test results for Ms. Parlet: Hgb 11.2 g/dL; BS 115, NF; dipstick urine negative for sugar, albumin (protein), leukocytes; pH 7; specific gravity 1.025. (*Note:* NF, nonfasting.)

PATIENT'S NAME	☐ FEMALE ☐ MALE Date of Birth: ___/___/___
DATE	PATIENT VISITS AND FINDINGS

ALLERGIC TO _____

PAGE _____ of _____

2. Below, fill in the results from the CLIA-waived testing performed during her visit.
(*Note:* To indicate that the glucose result was nonfasting, label as NF.)

FLOW SHEET

Name: *Louise Parlet*   **Date of Birth:** *07/04/1982* **Age:** *23*

Vital Signs Date:	05/01/07							
Weight	125 lbs							
Height	5 ft 5 in							
Temperature	98.2 F							
Pulse	72							
Respirations	16							
Blood Pressure	104/72							
Lab Tests Date:	05/01/07							
CBC								
RBC								
WBC								
HGB								
Hematocrit								
Alkaline Phosphatase								
Albumin								
Glucose								
Bilirubin total								
BUN								
Calcium								
Cholesterol								
Chloride								
CO2								
Creatinine								
Hb A1c								
LipidProfile								
LDL								
HDL								
Triglycerides								
SGGT								
SGOG/AST								
SGPT/ATL								
LDH								
T3								
T4								
T7								
TSH								
Triglycerides								
Total Protein								
Uric Acid								
Sodium								
Potassium								
Urinalysis								
Albumin								
Glucose								
PAPSmear								
PSA								
Other tests:								

3. Dr. Hayler received a partial report on Ms. Parlet's laboratory results today. Document the results in the blank Progress Notes below, using 5/01/2007 as the collection date. Include the following results: Hgb 10.6 g/dL; Hct 38%; RBC 4.2; WBC 5400; platelet count 200,000; pregnancy test positive; rubella titer 1:1 (assumed immune); ABO O; Rh+; PAP negative; Chlamydia negative.

PATIENT'S NAME	☐FEMALE ☐MALE Date of Birth: __/__/__
DATE	**PATIENT VISITS AND FINDINGS**

ALLERGIC TO _____

PAGE _____ of _____

4. Below, document the laboratory results from the Progress Notes onto the flow sheet.

FLOW SHEET

Name: *Louise Parlet*   **Date of Birth:** *07/04/1982* **Age:** *23*

Vital Signs Date:	05/01/07						
Weight	125 lbs						
Height	5 ft 5 in						
Temperature	98.2 F						
Pulse	72						
Respirations	16						
Blood Pressure	104/72						
Lab Tests Date:	05/01/07						
CBC							
RBC							
WBC							
HGB							
Hematocrit							
Alkaline Phosphatase							
Albumin							
Glucose							
Bilirubin total							
BUN							
Calcium							
Cholesterol							
Chloride							
CO2							
Creatinine							
Hb A1c							
LipidProfile							
LDL							
HDL							
Triglycerides							
SGGT							
SGOG/AST							
SGPT/ATL							
LDH							
T3							
T4							
T7							
TSH							
Triglycerides							
Total Protein							
Uric Acid							
Sodium							
Potassium							
Urinalysis							
Albumin							
Glucose							
PAPSmear							
PSA							
Other tests:							

5. Should any of Ms. Parlet's laboratory test results be highlighted for the physician for special attention? If so, which one(s)? (*Hint:* Refer to your answers in Exercise 2, question 4.)

Performing Blood Chemistry Testing

Reading Assignment: Chapter 51—Assisting in the Chemical Laboratory
- Quality Assurance and Quality Control

Chapter 54—Assisting in the Analysis of Blood
- Clinical Chemistry
- Blood Glucose Testing
- Cholesterol Testing

Patient: Rhea Davison

Learning Objectives:

- List the CLIA-waived chemistry tests commonly performed in a medical office.
- Name common blood chemistry tests performed in the medical office.
- Discuss the necessity of quality control for blood glucose tests in home and office testing.
- State the length of time to which fructosamine values correlate in regard to the patient's average glucose level.
- Identify the normal ranges of more commonly performed chemistry testing.
- Discuss the needed preparation for a fasting blood glucose or cholesterol test.
- Indicate which tests should be obtained as fasting chemistry tests when possible.
- State the patient teaching important in obtaining blood glucose tests using an Accu-Chek glucose meter.
- Describe the proper storage of blood glucose testing supplies.
- Complete the laboratory log for specimens being sent to an outside laboratory.
- Document the test results on a laboratory flow sheet and indicate those tests that need to be seen by the physician as soon as possible.

Overview:

In this lesson you will describe the collection and handling of some of the common CLIA-waived blood chemistry tests performed in the medical office. The normal range of blood chemistry results will be identified, and the ability to evaluate the test results will be emphasized. You will be expected to complete a laboratory log for specimens being sent to outside laboratories for testing. You will also document the return of the test results to the office. As the medical assistant, you will be asked to evaluate results that need immediate attention and those that can be seen by the physician at the end of the day. Rhea Davison is an established patient with a known history of diabetes mellitus. She has kept her diabetes well controlled until

349

her last visit. The physician is concerned that the glucose meter (glucometer) she is using at home may be providing inaccurate results, so you are asked to assist Ms. Davison in learning how to perform routine maintenance on the glucose meter.

Exercise 1

Writing Activity—Common Blood Chemistry Testing

  25 minutes

1. What is measured through blood chemistry testing?

2. Into which classification (complexity) of CLIA tests do most chemistry analyzers fall?

3. Name a few of the blood chemistry tests that are commonly performed in the medical office laboratory.

4. What preparation is needed for a fasting cholesterol test in the medical office?

5. What is the best appointment time for the patient to have a fasting cholesterol test? Why?

6. Express the blood glucose result that correlates with the glycosylated hemoglobin (HgbA1c) results.

7. What are some side effects that may occur in a patient who is having a glucose tolerance test?

8. What is the patient given to drink when having the glucose tolerance test?

9. If the physician orders a fructosamine test, how long will this correlate or "look back" at the results of the patient's glucose level?

Exercise 2

Online Activity—Patient Education for Quality Blood Glucose Tests

30 minutes

- Sign in to Mountain View Clinic.
- From the patient list, select **Rhea Davison**.

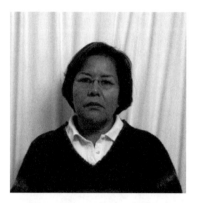

- On the office map, highlight and click on **Exam Room**.

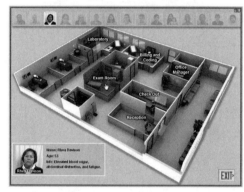

- In the Exam Room, click on **Exam Notes** to read the initial documentation of Ms. Davison's visit.
- Click on **Close** to return to the Exam Room.

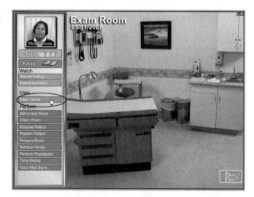

- Under the Watch heading, click on **Waived Testing** to view the video.
- Click **Close** at the end of the video to return to the Exam Room.

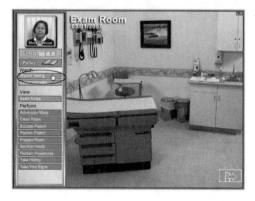

1. Now that you have read the Exam Notes and watched the video, why do you think that Dr. Meyer wants Ms. Davison to perform a glucose test using the equipment in the office?

- Remain in the Exam Room with Ms. Davison and select **Prepare Room** from the Perform menu.

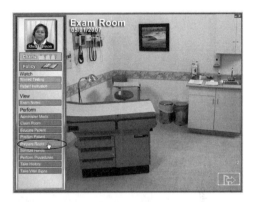

- Select the first item needed for Ms. Davison's visit from the alphabetical list and click **Add Item** to confirm your choice. Each item you add will appear in the Selected Supplies box.
- Repeat this step until you are satisfied you have everything you need from the list. Leave this window open as you answer the following questions. (*Reminder:* The Exam Notes are available in the bottom left corner of your screen if you need to refer to them.)

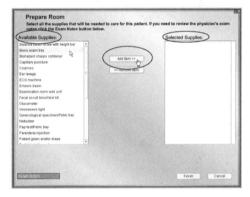

2. List the supplies needed by a medical assistant for blood glucose testing.

3. Which of the following supplies would be needed by Ms. Davison for performing quality control of the glucose testing equipment she currently uses at home? Select all that apply.

_____ Abnormal control sample

_____ Gloves

_____ Normal control

_____ Glucose meter

_____ Sterile wipes

_____ Container for sharps

_____ Glucose reagent strips

_____ Capillary lancet

➤ • Click **Finish** to return to the Exam Room.

4. Indicate whether each of the following statements is true or false.

a. _____ All chemistry test results are confined to only a single number for normal readings.

b. _____ Cholesterol and blood glucose may be CLIA-waived tests.

c. _____ To perform cholesterol and blood glucose testing in the medical office, the equipment must be CLIA-waived unless highly qualified personnel are available for the testing.

d. _____ At home, a patient should store equipment away from light and heat sources.

e. _____ The fructose tests provide a record of the average of the patient's glucose level for 5 months.

f. _____ Quality control is necessary for ensuring that chemistry test equipment is working properly.

g. _____ Blood chemistry testing is used for differential diagnoses.

h. _____ The equipment used by patients at home is CLIA-waived.

i. _____ All types of blood glucose equipment have the same instructions for use.

5. What information needs to be supplied to Ms. Davison about the collection of the specimen immediately following the capillary puncture?

6. What information should be supplied to Ms. Davison about the use of the glucose meter?

7. The medical assistant suggests that Ms. Davison ask the physician for a new glucose testing meter. Why do you think this is important?

8. In the Exam Notes, Ms. Davison reports having missed several doses of medication because of the inability to buy the medication. How would you expect this to affect the test results she obtained at home?

9. Would you expect Ms. Davison to have an increase in weight if she is following her prescribed diet? Explain your answer.

10. What information did Ms. Davison give about where she stores her glucose meter, and what affect may this have on the results of her tests?

 • Click the exit arrow to leave the Exam Room.

• If you wish to see your Prepare Room exercise results, click on **Look at Your Performance Summary** and compare your answers with those of the experts.

• To continue with this lesson, click on **Return to Map**.

• On the office map, click on **Check Out** to review the final documentation of Ms. Davison's visit.

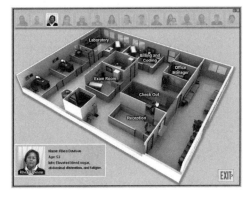

• Click on **Charts**.

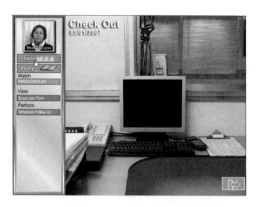

• Select **1-Progress Notes** from the drop-down menu under the **Patient Medical Information** tab.

• Read the results of today's blood glucose test and the testing that is to be done on the next day.

• Remain at the Check Out desk with Ms. Davison's Progress Notes open to answer the remaining questions in this exercise.

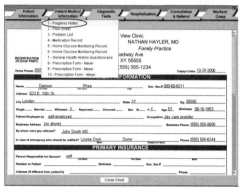

11. Is the test result for Ms. Davison's blood glucose obtained in the office within the limits expected when compared with the results from her home testing? Explain your answer.

12. Dr. Meyer ordered an HgbA1c. What information does this test provide? Why is this an important test for Dr. Meyer to use in treating Ms. Davison?

Exercise 3

Writing Activity—Quality Control with Blood Chemistry Testing

15 minutes

In this exercise you will use your knowledge to decide whether quality control has been accomplished.

1. Indicate whether each of the following statements is true or false.

   a. _____ Quality control for blood chemistry testing should be done no more than once a day.

   b. _____ When new reagent strips are opened, quality control sampling should occur.

   c. _____ Quality control samples have expiration dates.

   d. _____ Quality control samples may be used with any equipment.

   e. _____ Quality control is performed only so that the physician will have an accurate reading for comparison.

   f. _____ If the quality control samples are consistently inaccurate, the patient should try to repair the equipment used at home, because the patient is the person who best understands how that specific equipment works.

   g. _____ One method of checking for quality control of a machine in the medical office is to compare results obtained from a reference laboratory on a specific specimen with the results obtained on that same specimen in the office laboratory.

2. What is the significance if samples for quality control fall out of the control range?

3. If a patient questions the importance of performing quality control on a regular basis, what should you tell the patient?

Exercise 4

Online Activity—Preparing a Laboratory Log for Patient Specimens

10 minutes

1. Rhea Davison's specimens were sent to an outside laboratory (Quality Lab) the day following her appointment. Using her Progress Notes, prepare the laboratory log below for these tests. (*Note:* The requisition number has been filled in for you.)

Requisition Number	Date of Specimen Collected	Patient Name	Laboratory Test	Processing Laboratory	Initials: Specimen Collection	Date of Results Return	Initials: Results Return
112417							

Exercise 5

Online Activity—Adding Laboratory Results to the Flow Sheet

30 minutes

1. On the flow sheet on the next page, transfer the test results recorded in Ms. Davison's Progress Notes for 5/1/2007. Also add the following results, which were received by Dr. Meyer on 5/3/2007:

   - Blood chemistry: albumin 4.2; alkaline phosphatase 4; bilirubin 1.2; SGOT 14; calcium 7.2; chloride 98; creatinine 0.6; LDH 96; glucose 460; potassium 4.8; total protein 6.6; sodium 130; urea nitrogen 18; phosphorus 3.2
   - Thyroid profile: T4 10.8; T3 185; TSH 15.4
   - CA 125: 3.6
   - HgbA1c: 10

   After you have filled in the flow chart, compare Ms. Davison's results with the normal value ranges listed in the table provided on pages 1185 and 1186 of the Kinn's Medical Assistant 11e textbook. Place an asterisk (*) next to any of Ms. Davison's results that should be given prompt attention.

FLOW SHEET

Name: *Rhea Davison* _____ Date of Birth: *08/16/1953* Age: *53*

Vital Signs Date:	05/01/07							
Weight	152 lbs							
Height	5 ft 1 in							
Temperature	98.6 F							
Pulse	86							
Respirations	24							
Blood Pressure	144/86							
Lab Tests Date:								
CBC								
RBC								
WBC								
HGB								
Hematocrit								
Alkaline Phosphatase								
Albumin								
Glucose								
Bilirubin total								
BUN								
Calcium								
Cholesterol								
Chloride								
CO2								
Creatinine								
HgbA1c								
LipidProfile								
LDL								
HDL								
Triglycerides								
SGGT								
SGOT/AST								
SGPT/ATL								
LDH								
T3								
T4								
T7								
TSH								
Triglycerides								
Total Protein								
Urea Nitrogen								
Sodium								
Potassium								
Urinalysis								
Albumin								
Glucose								
PAPSmear								
PSA								
Other tests:								

Performing Immunology Testing

👓 **Reading Assignment:** Chapter 41—Assisting in Obstetrics and Gynecology
- Diagnostic Testing

Chapter 52—Assisting in the Analysis of Urine
- Urine Pregnancy Testing

Chapter 55—Assisting in Microbiology and Immunology
- Miscellaneous Microbiology Testing

Patients: Louise Parlet, Kevin McKinzie

Learning Objectives:

- Explain what information immunological tests can provide.
- Discuss what is meant by a false-negative result or false-positive result.
- Understand the importance of reading the package instructions prior to performing tests on a sample.
- Recognize when the antibody level is highest during an infection and when the antibody level starts to decline.
- Understand the importance of following directions for pregnancy testing.
- Describe the reaction that takes place in Mono testing.
- Document laboratory test results appropriately.

Overview:

In this lesson you will learn about the different types of immunology testing and the reasons this type of testing is used. A newly pregnant woman, Louise Parlet, provides blood and urine specimens for pregnancy and serology testing.

Exercise 1

Online Activity/Writing Activity—What Is Immunology Testing?

25 minutes

1. What information does immunological testing provide?

2. When does a person form antibodies?

3. Which of the following antigens can cause the production of antibodies? Use your critical thinking skills while answering this question and select all that could apply.

_____ Viruses

_____ Bacteria

_____ Cat dander

_____ Electricity

_____ Pollen

_____ Water

_____ Earthworms

_____ Wheat

_____ Eggs

_____ Nuts (tree or ground)

4. During which phase of a disease would the antibody level be the highest, and when does it start declining?

5. Which of the following types of specimens can be used for immunology testing? Select all that apply.

_____ Feces

_____ Blood

_____ Urine

_____ Sputum

6. Which of the following tests are based on an antigen-antibody reaction? Select all that apply.

_____ ABO blood typing

_____ QuickVue Mono test

_____ Hemoccult

_____ Sputum for acid-fast bacillus

_____ Syphilis titers

_____ VDRL

_____ Hepatitis titers

_____ CBC

_____ ASO test

7. Describe what is meant by a false-positive or false-negative test.

8. A false-negative result for immunology tests may be referred to as the _____

   _____.

9. What are the dangers of false-positive and false-negative test results? Apply critical thinking skills to answer this question.

10. Prior to performing any test, what should the medical assistant do once the test kit is opened?

11. Why is this step so important?

12. What is the name of the acute infectious disease that is also referred to as the "kissing disease"?

13. Patients of what age range are more frequently affected by mononucleosis?

14. What virus causes mononucleosis?

15. Discuss the antigen-antibody reaction in the Mono tests.

→ • Sign in to Mountain View Clinic.
 • From the patient list, select **Kevin McKinzie**.

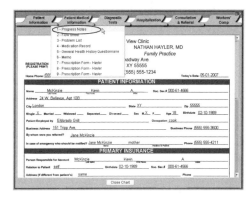

 • On the office map, highlight and click on **Check Out**.

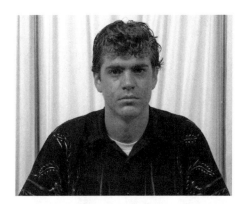

 • Click on **Charts** and then on the **Patient Medical Information** tab. Select **1-Progress Notes** from the drop-down menu and read the documentation from Mr. McKinzie's visit.

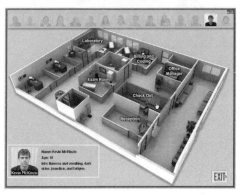

16. What was the result of Mr. McKinzie's QuickVue Mono test?

17. What type of specimen was used for this screening?

Exercise 2

Online Activity—Immunology Testing with Urine Pregnancy Testing

40 minutes

In this exercise you will work with Louise Parlet, a newly pregnant patient. She has performed a pregnancy test at home that was positive and has now come to the physician's office to verify the pregnancy.

1. The most common type of test used for pregnancy testing is the _____

   _____ _____ test.

2. What is the substance in urine that is present to show a positive pregnancy test?

3. When is the substance you identified in question 2 at its highest peak in plasma?

4. Identify whether each of the following statements is true or false.

   a. _____ hCG is first apparent as early as 1 week after implantation or 4 to 5 days before a missed menstrual period.

   b. _____ The level of hCG remains the same throughout pregnancy.

   c. _____ Most pregnancy tests take 20 minutes to perform.

d. _____ The best urine specimen to use for a pregnancy test is the first morning specimen.

e. _____ When properly used, urine pregnancy tests are only 75% effective.

f. _____ Pregnancy tests do not have built in "controls" to ensure that the test is performed correctly.

g. _____ If a pregnancy test is performed early in the pregnancy, the test should be repeated later to confirm the results.

- Sign in to Mountain View Clinic.
- From the patient list, select **Louise Parlet**.

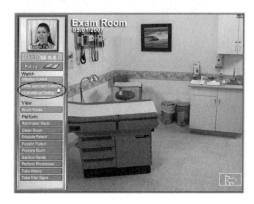

- On the office map, highlight and click on **Exam Room**.

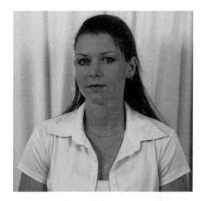

- Under the Watch heading, select **Urine Specimen Collection** to view the video.
- Click **Close** at the end of the video to return to the Exam Room.

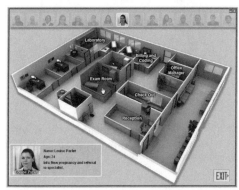

• Click on **CLIA-Waived Testing** to view the next video.
• Click **Finish** when you are finished watching the video.

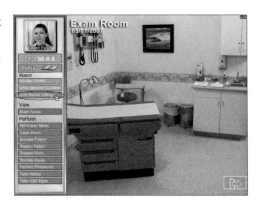

5. Ms. Parlet states that she has waited to void until her appointment. Why is the first-voided specimen more likely to provide accurate test results?

6. Why is it important for Ms. Parlet to collect a clean-catch midstream urine specimen?

7. The medical assistant who is training the student tells her that they do not keep a large inventory of pregnancy tests. What does she state as the reason for this?

8. How many drops of urine are suppose to be used in this particular test kit?

9. How long should the medical assistant wait before reading the results?

→ • Click on **Policy** to open the office Policy
  Manual.

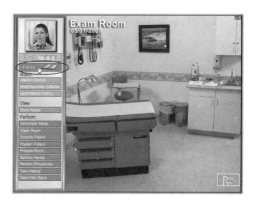

• In the search bar, type "standing orders" and
  click twice on the magnifying glass to access the
  relevant section.
• Read the policies on Pregnancy Testing that are
  part of the standing orders for this office.
• Click **Close Manual** to return to the
  Exam Room.

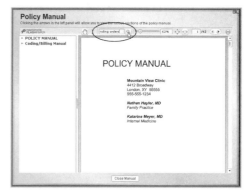

10. Why could the medical assistant perform a pregnancy test on Louise Parlet without a
    specific order from the physician?

11. According to the Exam Notes, what other immunology tests were ordered for Ms. Parlet?

→ • Click on the exit arrow to leave the Exam Room.
  • Click on **Return to Map** to return to the office map.

12. Joan Smith, born 7/28/1992, has come to Mountain View Clinic for a pregnancy test. Below, accurately document this test and its result, which was negative. This is the second testing of Joan Smith's urine using a QuickVue test. Use today's date and time. Be sure to sign the entry.

PATIENT'S NAME	☐FEMALE ☐MALE Date of Birth: __/__/__
DATE	PATIENT VISITS AND FINDINGS

ALLERGIC TO _____

PAGE _____ of _____

Wrapping Items for Sterilization

/Oℛⅅ **Reading Assignment:** Chapter 56—Surgical Supplies and Instruments
- Care and Handling of Instruments

Chapter 57—Surgical Asepsis and Assisting with Surgical Procedures
- Sterilization

Patient: Jose Imero

Learning Objectives:

- Identify the things to check for proper working order when instruments are received in the medical office.
- Understand the reasons for performing sanitization before sterilization.
- State the reason for using indicator strips in sterilization techniques and quality control.
- Identify the items needed for wrapping articles for sterilization.
- Sequence the steps required for wrapping items for sterilization.
- Match causes of improper sterilization with problems that will result if the proper technique is not followed.
- Discuss the storage requirements for items that have been autoclaved.

Overview:

In most cases, items that will come in contact with body tissues must be sterile. After a reusable item has been used for a patient, that item is sanitized and then prepared for sterilization. Preparation for sterilization of items that must remain sterile requires wrapping the item for storage after sterilization. A certain technique is necessary when wrapping items for the autoclave. We will review this technique in this lesson.

Exercise 1

Online Activity—Sanitizing and Sterilizing Equipment

 45 minutes

1. What are some of the things that you should check to ensure that new instruments are in good working order after you receive them from a supply company?

2. What does it mean to sanitize equipment?

3. When do instruments need to be sanitized?

4. If instruments cannot be sanitized immediately, what should you do?

5. What is the rationale for soaking instruments in this case?

6. What should the medical assistant wear while sanitizing sharp instruments?

- Sign in to Mountain View Clinic.
- From the patient list, select **Jose Imero**.

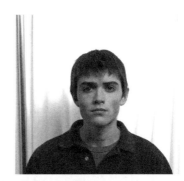

- On the office map, highlight **Exam Room** and click to enter the patient examination area.

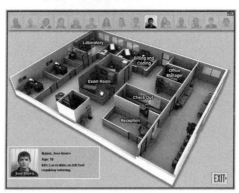

- In the Exam Room, click on **Sterilization Techniques** and watch the video. When the video is done, click **Finish**.

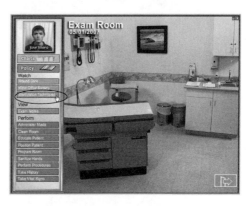

- Click on **Policy Manual**.

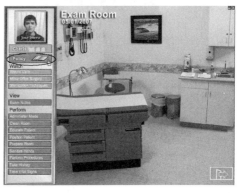

- Type "instruments" in the search bar and read about who is responsible for the sterilization of instruments.

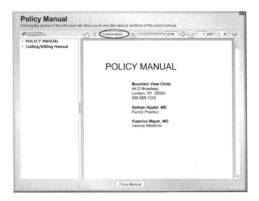

7. In the video, Charlie asks Danielle whether she has counted the instruments to see whether everything needed is on the tray. Why do you think he asked this question?

8. Why do you think Charlie asked whether the indicator strip was "in date"?

9. What is the reason for the indicator strip?

10. Which of the following supplies are needed when wrapping instruments and equipment for sterilization? Select all that apply.

_____ Wrapping paper or cloth/sterilization pouches

_____ Waterproof, felt-tipped pen

_____ Sterilization indicator

_____ Pencil

_____ Autoclave tape

11. If your autoclave tape has turned colors, does this indicate that the package is sterile? Support your answer.

12. Why is it important to make sure the wrapping material is an appropriate size for the item being wrapped?

13. Charlie told Danielle to begin with the wrapping material in a diamond shape. Why is this important when wrapping articles for sterilization?

14. Indicate whether each of the following statements is true or false.

a. _____ When instruments with movable parts are being wrapped, the joint should be closed to prevent moisture from adhering to the instrument and causing rust.

b. _____ When instruments with sharp edges are being wrapped, the edges should first be wrapped in gauze.

c. _____ The sterilization strip shows that the package has been sterilized.

d. _____ Autoclave tape indicates that the package is sterile.

e. _____ Any ballpoint pen is acceptable for labeling a package for the autoclave.

f. _____ The first fold made in wrapping an instrument should be the fold closest to your body at the bottom of the package.

15. Which of the following should appear on the label of a wrapped article for the autoclave? Select all that apply.

_____ Type of instrument or equipment found in the package

_____ Indicator strip inside

_____ Date of sterilization

_____ Initials of the person preparing the package

_____ Expiration date for the package

16. Match the columns below to show the correct sequence of steps in wrapping an instrument for autoclaving.

Action	Step Number
_____ Fold the top corner of the wrap toward the center and fold a tab.	a. Step 1
_____ Fold the bottom corner of the wrapping material toward the center and fold a tab.	b. Step 2
_____ Place the autoclave tape across the outside corner.	c. Step 3
_____ Flip the instrument in the wrap until it is a neat package.	d. Step 4
_____ Fold each side of the wrap into the center, leaving a tab on each side.	e. Step 5

17. Below are problems that may be experienced when autoclaving instruments. Match each problem with its possible cause.

Problem	Causes
_____ Ebullition	a. Too rapid exhausting of the chamber
_____ Corroded instruments	b. Vacuum in the chamber
_____ Damp linens	c. Dirty chamber
_____ Steam leakage	d. Poor cleaning
_____ Stained linens	e. Corrosion or soil in the joint
_____ Spotted or stained instruments	f. Clogged chamber drain
_____ Chamber door not opening	g. Mineral deposits on instruments
_____ Instruments with soft hinges or joints	h. Worn gasket

18. Once the medical assistant has sterilized the instruments, how should they be stored?

LESSON 33

Assisting with Minor Office Surgery

👓 **Reading Assignment:** Chapter 56—Surgical Supplies and Instruments
Chapter 57—Surgical Asepsis and Assisting with Surgical Procedures
- Surgical Procedures
- Assisting with Surgical Procedures
- Wound Care

Patients: Jose Imero, Tristan Tsosie

Learning Objectives:

- Identify instruments by their use or function.
- Discuss the correct procedure for preparing the patient for suturing of a laceration.
- Describe the importance of infection control and a sterile aseptic technique with minor surgery.
- Understand the appropriate disposal of biohazardous materials when performing wound care.
- Read and understand progress notes pertaining to surgery and suture removal.
- Discuss the need for patient education following suturing of a laceration and suture removal.
- Chart entries pertaining to minor office surgery and suture removal.
- Apply critical thinking skills in regard to patient education related to minor office surgery.

Overview:

This lesson focuses on the medical assistant's role in assisting the physician with minor office surgery. You will observe and evaluate the medical assistant's preparation of patient Jose Imero for a suturing of lacerations. Another patient, Tristan Tsosie, has a laceration that needs suture removal. The necessary steps for this will be presented and evaluated.

Exercise 1

Online Activity—Assisting with Minor Office Surgery

 45 minutes

- Sign in to Mountain View Clinic.
- From the patient list, select **Jose Imero**.

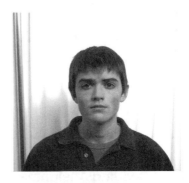

- On the office map, highlight and click on **Exam Room**.

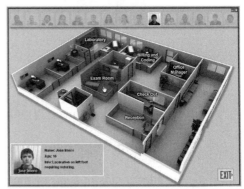

- Click on **Exam Notes** to read the documentation regarding Jose's visit. Note the procedures he is to have performed during his examination. Also review patient instructions. Click **Finish** to return to the Exam Room.

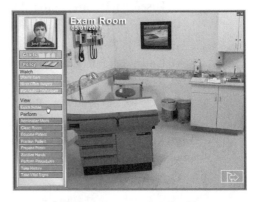

- Under the Perform heading, select **Prepare Room** to select the supplies needed for Jose's visit. (*Note:* You can reopen the Exam Notes for reference as you make your selections.)

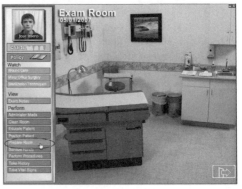

- Select the first item needed for Jose's visit from the alphabetical list and click **Add Item** to confirm your choice. The items you select will appear in the Selected Supplies column.
- Repeat this step until you are satisfied you have everything you need from the list.
- Do not close this window. Keep the Prepare Room wizard open as you continue with the lesson.

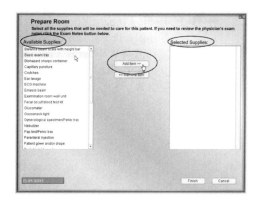

- In the Prepare Room wizard, click on **Wound Care** in the list of Available Supplies and review the contents on the tray shown in the photo.

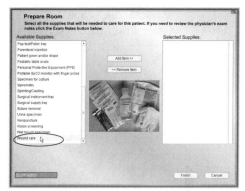

1. List the supplies (in any order) provided for wound care as shown in the photograph and explain why each is needed.

Supplied Item	Reason for Use

• In the Prepare Room wizard, select **Surgical Supply Tray** from the list of Available Supplies and review the tray's contents as shown in the photograph.

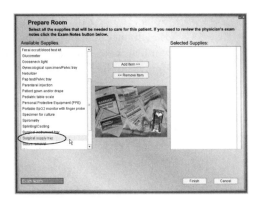

2. What disposable supplies are found on the supply tray that will be needed for the suturing of Jose's foot? (*Note:* You can check your answers when you watch the video later in this exercise.)

(1)

(2)

(3)

(4)

(5)

(6)

(7)

 • Next, click on **Surgical Instrument Tray** in the Available Supplies list. Again, review the tray's contents as shown in the photograph.

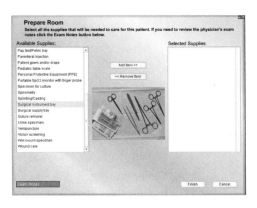

3. What instruments and supplies are found on the tray that could possibly be used for suturing Jose's foot?

4. In the video that you will be watching, Dr. Hayler will specifically state that he is going to probe Jose's wound for possible foreign objects. With that information, what sterile materials necessary for preparing to suture a laceration are missing from the surgical instrument tray?

5. Match each of the following surgical instruments with its use or description.

Instrument	Use or Description
_____ Scalpel	a. Used to find foreign objects in a wound
_____ Forceps	b. Used for grasping and squeezing
_____ Operating scissors	c. Used to open orifices
_____ Hemostats	d. Have straight sharp blades for cutting through tissue
_____ Needle holders	e. Small surgical knife used to cut through tissue
_____ Retractors	f. Used to pull back tissue and skin
_____ Speculum	g. Forceps-like instrument used to hold circular needles
_____ Suture scissors	h. Used to clamp blood vessels and to hold tissue
_____ Probe	i. Forceps with straight sharp points for removing foreign objects from wounds
_____ Splinter forceps	j. Scissors used to cut sutures

- Click **Finish** to close the Prepare Room wizard and return to the Exam Room.
- Under the Watch heading, click on **Wound Care** to view the video.
- At the end of the video, click **Close** to return to the Exam Room (*Remember:* You can click on the play button if you wish to replay the video.)

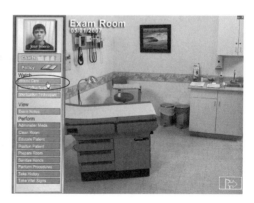

6. Why do you think the red bag was taped onto the Mayo stand?

7. Why did Charlie place a protective sheet under Jose's foot?

- If you have not already closed this video, click **Close** now.
- Under Watch, select **Minor Office Surgery** to watch the next video.
- While watching this video, look for a distinct break in sterile technique.

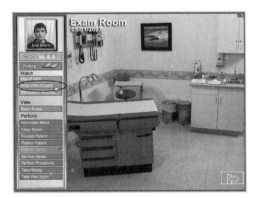

8. What is the break in sterile technique that Charlie allows to happen?

9. Why was it important that Charlie pass the suture material around the surgical tray?

10. Apply critical thinking skills and your knowledge from the chapter to indicate whether each of the following statements is true or false.

a. _____ The medical assistant is responsible for supplying a light source when assisting with minor surgery.

b. _____ When setting a sterile field, the entire area is considered sterile.

c. _____ When preparing a tray for suturing during minor surgery, it is most time efficient to place the instruments in the order of use.

d. _____ The medical assistant should pay close attention as the surgery is being performed so he or she can anticipate anything with which the physician will need assistance.

e. _____ Once a minor surgery suture tray has been set, the medical assistant cannot add instruments or supplies to the tray.

f. _____ Surgical scissors may have sharp blades, blunt blades, or a combination of the two.

g. _____ When assisting with minor surgery, the medical assistant must always use sterile gloves.

h. _____ The application of sterile gloves requires a different technique from the application of nonsterile gloves.

i. _____ When pouring a solution onto a sterile field, the medical assistant should first pour the solution over the lip of the container into a waste receptacle container that is not on the sterile field and then discard it; the solution should then be poured into the sterile container on the sterile field (this applies to containers that do not have a double-cap system).

j. _____ When opening a sterile pack, the flap closest to you should be opened first.

k. _____ Suture material is always the same for each wound and each physician.

l. _____ Suture material comes in absorbable and nonabsorbable types.

m. _____ Absorbable suture is usually used for deep incisions or lacerations that require inner layers of sutures to close the wound.

n. _____ Nonabsorbable suture is usually used for deep tissue.

o. _____ Suture material comes in varying sizes, lengths, and absorbability.

p. _____ Skin may be closed with staples and adhesive skin closures.

q. _____ Selection of suture material depends on the site, length, and depth of the wound.

r. _____ According to the chart notes, Jose had 16 sutures placed in his foot.

11. What instructions did Dr. Hayler give Jose as he was suturing his laceration?

12. Why did Dr. Hayler tell Jose to use the crutches?

Critical Thinking Question

13. Identify some of the other reasons patients must be given instructions to follow when they have had an area sutured.

14. What was one other measure Dr. Hayler took to prevent Jose from getting an infection? (*Hint:* You may wish to reopen the Exam Notes in the Exam Room.)

15. What other instructions were given to the patient according to the Exam Notes?

 • Click **Close** and then click the exit arrow to leave the Exam Room.
   • Click **Return to Map**.

Exercise 2

 Online Activity—Assisting with Suture Removal

 20 minutes

Your instructor may indicate that watching the video is an optional assignment. In an earlier lesson, we watched Tristan Tsosie's wound care video and prepared his room for wound care.

• From the patient list, select **Tristan Tsosie**.
  (*Note:* If you have exited the program, sign in again to Mountain View Clinic and select Tristan Tsosie from the patient list.)

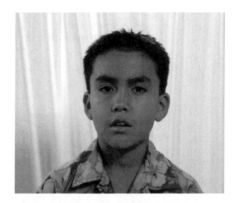

• On the office map, highlight and click on **Exam Room**.

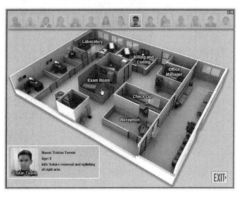

→ • Under Perform, click on **Prepare Room** to select the supplies needed for Tristan's visit.

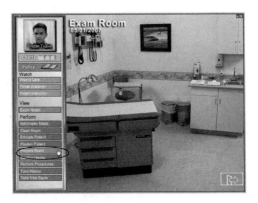

• From the list of Available Supplies, select **Suture Removal** and review the tray's contents as shown in the photo.

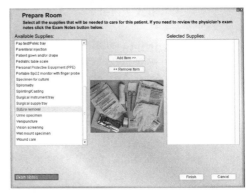

1. List the items shown on the tray.

2. Tristan had a wound culture taken. When should the cleansing of the stitches or wound take place?

- Click **Finish** to close the Prepare Room wizard.
- Under Watch, click **Wound Care** and watch the video. (*Note:* Your instructor may have assigned this in an earlier lesson, but watch the video to refresh your memory and answer the following questions.)
- Click **Close** when you are finished viewing the video.

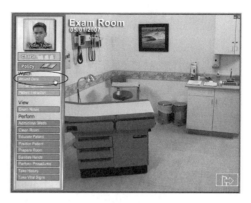

3. When the medical assistant was preparing Tristan for the removal of sutures, Tristan asked whether the procedure would hurt. Should the medical assistant have answered the question before continuing with the procedure, or was it effective communication to ignore the question at that point?

4. Indicate whether each of the following statements is true or false. Remember to use critical thinking skills in addition to your knowledge from the reading assignment.

   a. _____ Before removing sutures, the medical assistant should obtain the permission of the physician.

   b. _____ If the wound appears to gape open during suture removal and the physician has stated that all sutures should be removed, the medical assistant should continue to remove the sutures.

   c. _____ When sutures are being removed, the patient should be placed in a comfortable position to prevent injury or unnecessary discomfort.

   d. _____ Following injury, all sutures will be ready to be removed at the same time.

   e. _____ The size and location of the wound are important factors that the physician will take into consideration when instructing the patient when to return to the office for suture removal.

   f. _____ All sutures may be removed using the same size suture scissors and forceps, regardless of the location of the sutures.

g. _____ When cleansing the area before removing the sutures, the skin should be thoroughly cleansed and any dry exudate should be removed.

h. _____ When removing sutures, it is not important to count the sutures removed, since you need to remove only those you can see.

- Click on **Prepare Room** (under Perform) and select the first item needed for Tristan's visit from the alphabetical list and click **Add Item** to confirm your choice. The items you select will appear in the Selected Supplies column.

- Repeat this step until you are satisfied you have everything you need from the list. (*Note:* The Exam Notes are available if you need to refer to them.)

- Click **Finish** to return to the Exam Room.

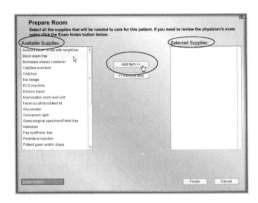

- In the Exam Room, select **Clean Room** (under Perform) and select the necessary steps to be taken at the end of Tristan's visit.

- Click **Finish** to return to the Exam Room.

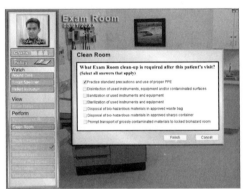

5. Why was it important for Tristan to keep his arm covered and splinted as the physician instructed?

6. Below, document the removal of sutures from a clean wound on Tristan Tsosie's leg. The sutures were inserted 6 days earlier. Be sure to document that the physician, Dr. Hayler, has observed the sutures and has told you to remove these seven sutures. Also document the dressing of the wound following removal and that the patient did not seem to have any problems. Use today's date for the documentation and your initials for the entry.

PATIENT'S NAME	☐ FEMALE ☐ MALE Date of Birth: / /
DATE	PATIENT VISITS AND FINDINGS

ALLERGIC TO _____

_____ PAGE _____ of _____

- Click the exit arrow to get to the Summary Menu.
- Select **Look at Your Performance Summary** to compare your answers with those of the experts.
- Select **Return to Map** to move on to the next lesson or select **Exit** to exit the program.

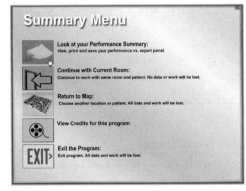